Advanced Buteyko Breathing Exercises

Artour Rakhimov

Dr. Artour Rakhimov

Copyright ©2013 Artour Rakhimov.

All rights reserved.

This book is copyrighted. It is prohibited to copy, lend, adapt, electronically transmit, or transmit by any other means or methods without prior written approval from the author. However, the book may be borrowed by family members.

Disclaimer

The content provided herein is for information purposes only and not intended to diagnose, treat, cure or prevent cystic fibrosis or any other chronic disease. Always consult your doctor or health care provider before making any medical decisions). The information herein is the sole opinion of Dr. Artour Rakhimov and does not constitute medical advice. These statements have not been evaluated by Ontario Ministry of Health. Although every effort has been made to ensure the accuracy of the information herein, Dr. Artour Rakhimov accepts no responsibility or liability and makes no claims, promises, or guarantees about the accuracy, completeness, or adequacy of the information provided herein and expressly disclaims any liability for errors and omissions herein.

Advanced Buteyko Breathing Exercises

Table of content

Introduction 6
CHAPTER 1. BODY O2 TEST OR CP TEST AND MORNING CP 8
   1.1 How to do the CP test 8
   1.2 Usual CP numbers in sick people 10
   1.3 Usual CP numbers in healthy and ordinary people 13
   1.4 How and why the morning CP is a crucial health test 18
CHAPTER 2. DIAPHRAGMATIC BREATHING 22
   2.1 Why do we need diaphragmatic breathing? 22
   2.2 How to test your own breathing technique 24
   2.3 Causes of diaphragm dysfunction and chest breathing in modern people 25
   2.4 How to restore function to the diaphragm 24/7? 27
   2.5 Specific techniques with diaphragmatic breathing: exercise with books 28
   2.6 Diaphragmatic breathing technique with belts 29
   2.7 Magnesium can be a key factor for some people 32
   2.8 Advanced diaphragmatic breathing exercises for unblocking the diaphragm 33
   2.9 Importance of posture for diaphragmatic breathing 34
CHAPTER 3. RESTRICTIONS, LIMITS, AND TEMPORARY CONTRAINDICATIONS ... 37
   3.1 Heart disease, migraine headaches, and panic attacks 38
   3.2 Presence of transplanted organs 40
   3.3 Breathing exercises during pregnancy 41
   3.4 Brain traumas and acute bleeding injuries 42
   3.5 Blood clots 43
   3.6 Acute stages (exacerbations) and life-threatening conditions 44
   3.7 Loss of CO2 sensitivity 44
   3.8 Breathing exercises for underweight (or low weight) people 45
   3.9 Breathing exercises and prescribed medical drugs 46
CHAPTER 4. BUTEYKO EXERCISES FOR BEGINNERS 48
   4.1 Preliminary requirements for learning Buteyko breathing exercises 48
   4.2 The simple mechanics of normal breathing at rest or how the diaphragm works 52
   4.3 Breathing patterns 53
   4.4 Buteyko Table of Health Zones 56
   4.5 Feeling the breath and learning how to relax 57
   4.6 Relaxing the diaphragm (Buteyko relaxed breathing exercise) 60
   4.7 Buteyko reduced breathing exercise with light air hunger 62
   4.8 Using reduced breathing for symptoms, sleep, and bowel movements .. 68

4.9 Your daily log for breathing exercises and how to fill it 69
4.10 Structure and effects of one breathing session 73
4.11 Some questions and answers about breathing exercises and the CP test 79
4.12 Structure of the program of Buteyko breathing exercises 85
4.13 "Two hundred breath holds" 89
4.14 Use of imagery 90
4.15 Simple visualization applied to muscle groups 91
4.16 Imagery of scenes for better relaxation 93

CHAPTER 5. BREATH HOLDS AND MAXIMUM PAUSES: HEALTH EFFECTS AND USES 96
5.1 Maximum pauses, long breath holds and modern Buteyko teachers 96
5.2 Effects of maximum pauses and long breath holds on arteries and arterioles 97
5.3 When and for whom long breath holds can cause problems 98
5.4 Cases with severe bleeding 102
5.5 Loss of CO2 sensitivity 103
5.6 Other possible negative effects of maximum pauses or long breath holds 104
5.7 Common positive effects of maximum pauses or long breath holds 105
5.8 How to check your reactions to maximum pauses and long breath holds 106
5.9 Summary of effects of breath holds 107

CHAPTER 6. INTENSIVE BUTEYKO BREATHING EXERCISES 108
6.1 How to create moderate or strong levels of air hunger 108
6.2 A breathing session with moderate intensity 109
6.3 Intensive breathing sessions (with a strong air hunger) 113
6.4 AMP and very intensive breathing sessions 115
6.5 Sessions with variable breath holds and air hunger 116
6.6 The "click effect" 117
6.7 Overtraining due to breathing exercises 118
6.8 Summary of intensive breathing exercises 121

CHAPTER 7. TREATMENT OF BLUNTED AND LOST CO2 SENSITIVITY 122
7.1 Differences between blunted and lost CO2 sensitivity 122
7.2 Treatment of blunted CO2 sensitivity 123
7.3 Restoration of normal heart rate 124
7.4 Restoration of normal CO2 sensitivity 126

CHAPTER 8. BREATHING EXERCISES DURING PHYSICAL ACTIVITY 128
8.1 Restrictions and limitations 128

8.2 Breathing techniques during exercise for people with various CP ranges 130
8.3 Exercise 1. Breath holds and reduced breathing during physical exercise 132
8.4 Exercise 2. "Steps for Adults" 133
8.5 Breathing devices for physical exercise... 138
CONCLUSIONS 141
ABOUT THE AUTHOR: DR. ARTOUR RAKHIMOV 143

Dr. Artour Rakhimov

Introduction

Buteyko breathing exercises have been evolving since the 1960's, when Dr. Konstantin Buteyko, MD, PhD, developed his first respiratory technique. It is known as the "Buteyko reduced breathing exercise" and it forms the foundation for various subsequent Buteyko exercises. For example, some years after the invention of this exercise, Dr. Buteyko and his colleagues added breath holds as a part of his exercises. During the following decades, there were various changes in the structure of Buteyko exercises. These changes are mainly related to duration of a single breathing session and types and frequencies of applied breath holds.

Throughout the last 50 years, over 150 Soviet and Russian medical professionals (mostly family physicians or general practitioners) have applied Buteyko respiratory exercises on thousands of their patients. In total, well over 300,000 people learned these exercises from these doctors. Obviously, they accumulated rich clinical experience in this area. For example, it was discovered that people with panic attacks and hypertension can't get health benefits while practicing more common forms of Buteyko exercises developed for people with asthma, bronchitis, and diabetes.

In addition, they found that there are experience-related differences. Learners or novices get maximum health benefits and the highest results for the body oxygen test, if they practice breathing exercises for learners. The majority of advanced students, though, are able to get maximum benefits from advanced Buteyko breathing exercises.

While the title of this book suggests only advanced exercises, it includes those respiratory exercises that were designed and have been used for novices. In other words, the book includes initial, intermediate and advanced exercises developed and used by Dr. Buteyko and his medical colleagues.

Bear in mind, that according to experience of Soviet and Russian doctors, a breathing student needs to learn and understand certain physiological facts and laws before starting breathing retraining.

Advanced Buteyko Breathing Exercises

These physiological facts and laws include:
- Clinical norms for breathing at rest
- Breathing parameters in people with chronic diseases
- Why overbreathing (or breathing more than the medical norm) reduces O2 delivery to body cells
- Main qualities and effects of carbon dioxide on the human body
- Why slower and easier breathing at rest increases body oxygenation (even if you breathe 2-3 times less than the medical norm).

While teaching hundreds of Western students, I have discovered that additional education in relation to breathing during sleep and exercise, as well as certain other facts and laws, greatly assists better learning and improves their final results. This book outlines these additional factors and provides detailed descriptions of Buteyko breathing exercises from the initial to advanced level.

Dr. Artour Rakhimov

Chapter 1. Body O2 test or CP test and morning CP

"All chronic pain, suffering and diseases are caused from a lack of oxygen at the cell level."
Prof. A.C. Guyton, MD, The Textbook of Medical Physiology*

* World's most widely used medical textbook of any kind
* World's best-selling physiology book

1.1 How to do the CP test

The DIY body-O2 test is a very accurate health test. Clinical experience of Soviet and Russian Buteyko doctors shows that this test is the most representational in relation to the health state of people with health symptoms and/or chronic diseases. This test is also called the CP (Control Pause).

CP (Control Pause) = Body O2 test

You can eat tons of supplements and super-foods, drink canisters of herbal drinks, have hundreds of colonic irrigations, and practice (modern) yoga for many hours every day, but if your body oxygen level remains the same, you will suffer from the same symptoms and require the same dosage of medication.

Let us now consider the test itself.

Sit down and rest for 5-7 minutes. Completely relax all your muscles, including the breathing muscles. This relaxation produces natural spontaneous exhalation (breathing out). Pinch your nose closed at the end of this exhalation and count your BHT (breath holding time) in seconds. Keep the nose pinched until you experience the first desire to breathe. Practice shows that this first desire appears together with an involuntary push of the diaphragm or swallowing movement in the throat. (Your body warns you, "Enough!") If you release the nose and start breathing at this time,

Advanced Buteyko Breathing Exercises

you can resume your usual breathing pattern (in the same way as you were breathing prior to the test).

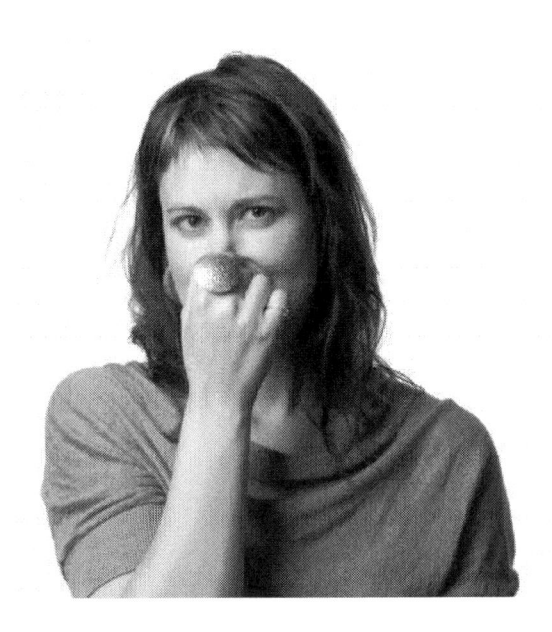

Do not extend breath holding too long, trying to increase the control pause. You should not gasp for air or open your mouth when you release your nose. Your breathing after the test should be the same as before the test, as it is shown here:

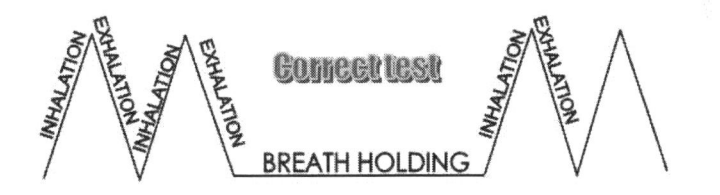

The test should be easy and not cause you any stress. This stress-free test should not interfere with your breathing. Here is the most common mistake that I have observed in thousands of people:

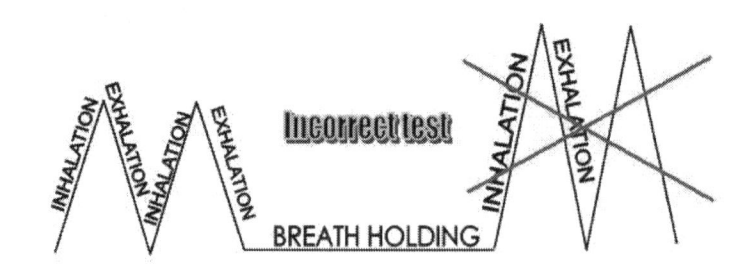

It is common for novices to make this mistake. However, if you repeat this test 3-4 times (with about 3-4 minutes of rest between successive attempts), you will find out that you can do the test correctly. Or, if you overdo the test by, let's say, 2-3 seconds, you need to subtract these 2-3 seconds in order to define your real CP.

Warning. Some, not all, people with migraine headaches, panic attacks, and heart disease, especially hypertension, may experience negative symptoms minutes later after this light version of the test. If this happens, they should temporary avoid this test.

Practical suggestion. Measure your CP throughout the day so that you know your usual CP dynamic. It will help you to find out those adverse lifestyle factors or environmental parameters that are most destructive for your health.

1.2 Usual CP numbers in sick people

"If a person breath-holds after a normal exhalation,
it takes about 40 seconds before breathing commences"
From the textbook "Essentials of exercise physiology"
McArdle W.D., Katch F.I., Katch V.L. (2nd edition);
Lippincott, Williams and Wilkins, London 2000, p.252.

More detailed results of these Western medical and physiological research studies are summarized in these Tables.

Body-oxygen test in sick people (13 medical studies)

Advanced Buteyko Breathing Exercises

Condition	N. of subjects	Body O2	Reference
Hypertension	95	12 s	Ayman et al, 1939
Neurocirculatory asthenia	54	16 s	Friedman, 1945
Anxiety states	62	20 s	Mirsky et al, 1946
Class 1 heart patients	16	16 s	Kohn & Cutcher, 1970
Class 2-3 heart patients	53	13 s	Kohn & Cutcher, 1970
Pulmonary emphysema	3	8 s	Kohn & Cutcher, 1970
Functional heart disease	13	5 s	Kohn & Cutcher, 1970
Asymptomatic asthmatics	7	20 s	Davidson et al, 1974
Asthmatics with symptoms	13	11 s	Perez-Padilla et al, 1989
Panic attack	14	11 s	Zandbergen et al, 1992

Condition	N. of subjects	Body O2	Reference
Anxiety disorders	14	16 s	Zandbergen et al, 1992
Outpatients	25	17 s	Gay et al, 1994
Inpatients	25	10 s	Gay et al, 1994
COPD + congen heart failure	7	8 s	Gay et al, 1994
12 heavy smokers	12	8 s	Gay et al, 1994
Panic disorder	23	16 s	Asmudson & Stein, 1994
Obstructive sleep apnea	30	20 s	Taskar et al, 1995
Successful lung transplant	9	23 s	Flume et al, 1996
Successful heart transplant	8	28 s	Flume et al, 1996
Outpatients with COPD	87	8 s	Marks et al, 1997
Asthma	55	14 s	Nannini et al, 2007

Note. These results were adjusted to the breath-holding test done after exhalation and only until first stress since many studies used different tests: some of them were done after full inhalation, with 3 large breaths (before the test), etc. For details of these adjustments, visit NormalBreathing.com. The same adjustments were used for the next CP Table.

We can see that sick people gave less than 20 seconds for the CP test, and that the CP test correlates with the severity of their health problems.

References (in the same order)

Ayman D, Goldshine AD, The breath-holding test. A simple standard stimulus of blood pressure, Archives of Intern Medicine 1939, 63; p. 899-906.

Friedman M, Studies concerning the aetiology and pathogenesis of neurocirculatory asthenia III. The cardiovascular manifestations of neurocirculatory asthenia, Am Heart J 1945; 30, 378-391.

Mirsky I A, Lipman E, Grinker R R, Breath-holding time in anxiety state, Federation proceedings 1946; 5: p. 74.

Kohn RM & Cutcher B, Breath-holding time in the screening for rehabilitation potential of cardiac patients, Scand J Rehabil Med 1970; 2(2): p. 105-107.

Davidson JT, Whipp BJ, Wasserman K, Koyal SN, Lugliani R, Role of the carotid bodies in breath-holding, New England Journal of Medicine 1974 April 11; 290(15): p. 819-822.

Perez-Padilla R, Cervantes D, Chapela R, Selman M, Rating of breathlessness at rest during acute asthma: correlation with spirometry and usefulness of breath-holding time, Rev Invest Clin 1989 Jul-Sep; 41(3): p. 209-213.

Zandbergen J, Strahm M, Pols H, Griez EJ, Breath-holding in panic disorder, Compar Psychiatry 1992 Jan-Feb; 33(1): p. 47-51.

Gay SB, Sistrom C1L, Holder CA, Suratt PM, Breath-holding capability of adults. Implications for spiral computed tomography, fast-acquisition magnetic resonance imaging, and angiography, Invest Radiol 1994 Sep; 29(9): p. 848-851.

Asmundson GJ & Stein MB, Triggering the false suffocation alarm in panic disorder patients by using a voluntary breath-holding procedure, Am J Psychiatry 1994 Feb; 151(2): p. 264-266.

Taskar V, Clayton N, Atkins M, Shaheen Z, Stone P, Woodcock A, Breath-holding time in normal subjects, snorers, and sleep apnea patients, Chest 1995 Apr; 107(4): p. 959-962.

Flume PA, Eldridge FL, Edwards LJ, Mattison LE, Relief of the 'air hunger' of breathholding. A role for pulmonary stretch receptors, Respir Physiol 1996 Mar; 103(3): p. 221-232.

Marks B, Mitchell DG, Simelaro JP, Breath-holding in healthy and pulmonary-compromised populations: effects of hyperventilation and oxygen inspiration, J Magn Reson Imaging 1997 May-Jun; 7(3): p. 595-597.

Nannini LJ, Zaietta GA, Guerrera AJ, Varela JA, Fernandez AM, Flores DM, Breath-holding test in subjects with near-fatal asthma. A new index for dyspnea perception, Respiratory Medicine 2007, 101; p.246–253.

1.3 Usual CP numbers in healthy and ordinary people

CPs in healthy and normal subjects

Types of people investigated	Number of subjects	Control Pause, s	References
US aviators	319	41 s	Schneider, 1919
Fit instructors	22	46 s	Flack, 1920
Home defense pilots	24	49 s	Flack, 1920
British candidates	23	47 s	Flack, 1920
US candidates	7	45 s	Flack, 1920
Delivery pilots	27	39 s	Flack, 1920
Pilots trained for scouts	15	42 s	Flack, 1920
Min requir. for flying	-	34 s	Flack, 1920
Normal subjects	20	39 s	Schneider, 1930
Normal subjects	30	23 s	Friedman, 1945
Normal subjects	7	44 s	Ferris et al, 1946
Normal subjects	22	33 s	Mirsky et al, 1946
Aviation students	48	36 s	Karpovich, 1947
Normal subjects	80	28 s	Rodbard, 1947
Normal subjects	3	41 s	Stroud, 1959
Normal subjects	16	16 s	Kohn & Cutcher, 1970

Advanced Buteyko Breathing Exercises

Normal subjects	6	28 s	Davidson et al, 1974
Normal subjects	16	22 s	Stanley et al, 1975
Normal subjects	7	29 s	Gross et al, 1976
Normal subjects	6	36 s	Bartlett, 1977
Normal subjects	9	33 s	Mukhtar et al, 1986
Normal subjects	20	36 s	Morrissey et al, 1987
Normal subjects	14	25 s	Zandbergen et al, 1992
Normal subjects	26	21 s	Asmudson & Stein, 1994
Normal subjects	30	36 s	Taskar et al, 1995
Normal subjects	76	25 s	McNally & Eke, 1996
Normal subjects	8	32 s	Sasse et al, 1996
Normal subjects	10	38 s	Flume et al, 1996
Normal subjects	31	29 s	Marks et al, 1997
Normal males	36	29 s	Joshi et al, 1998
Normal females	33	23 s	Joshi et al, 1998
Healthy subjects	20	38 s	Morooka et al, 2000
Normal subjects	6	30 s	Bosco et al, 2004
Normal subjects	19	30 s	Mitrouska et al, 2007
Healthy subjects	14	34 s	Andersson et al, 2009

Generally, we see that the CPs for modern normal subjects are about 20-30 seconds, while people living during first decades of the 20th century had about 40-50 seconds.

References (in the same order)

Schneider, 1919 - Observations were made in 1919, published in Schneider, 1930, see below.

Flack M, Some simple tests of physical efficiency, Lancet 1920; 196: p. 210-212.

Schneider EC, Observation on holding the breath, Am J Physiol, 1930, 94, p. 464-470.

Friedman M, Studies concerning the aetiology and pathogenesis of neurocirculatory asthenia III. The cardiovascular manifestations of neurocirculatory asthenia, Am Heart J 1945; 30, p. 378-391.

Ferris EB, Engel GL, Stevens CD, Webb J, Voluntary breathholding, III. The relation of the maximum time of breathholding to the oxygen and carbon dioxide tensions of arterial blood, with a note on its clinical and physiological significance, J Clin Invest 1946, 25: 734-743.

Mirsky I A, Lipman E, Grinker R R, Breath-holding time in anxiety state, Federation proceedings 1946; 5: p. 74.

Karpovich PV, Breath holding as a test of physical endurance, Am J Physiol, 1947, 149: p. 720-723

Rodbard S, The effect of oxygen, altitude and exercise on breath-holding time, Am J Physiol 1947, 150: p. 142-148.

Stroud RC, Combined ventilatory and breath-holding evaluation of sensitivity to respiratory gases, J Appl Physiol 1959, 14: p. 353-356.

Kohn RM & Cutcher B, Breath-holding time in the screening for rehabilitation potential of cardiac patients, Scand J Rehabil Med 1970; 2(2): p. 105-107.

Davidson JT, Whipp BJ, Wasserman K, Koyal SN, Lugliani R, Role of the carotid bodies in breath-holding, New England Journal of Medicine 1974 April 11; 290(15): p. 819-822.

Stanley NN, Cunningham EL, Altose MD, Kelsen SG, Levinson RS, Cherniack NS, Evaluation of breath holding in hypercapnia as a simple clinical test of respiratory chemosensitivity, Thorax 1975 Jun; 30(3): p. 337-343.

Gross PM, Whipp BJ, Davidson JT, Koyal SN, Wasserman K, Role of carotid bodies in the heart rate response to breath holding in man. J of Amer Physiol 1976, 41 (3); p. 336-339.

Bartlett D, Effects of Valsalva and Mueller maneuvers on breath-holding time, J Appl Physiol: Respiratory, Environ. & Exercise Physiol 1977 May, 42(5): p. 717-721.

Mukhtar MR, Patrick JM, Ventilatory drive during face immersion in man, J. Physiol. 1986, 370; p. 13-24.

Morrissey SC, Keohane K, Coote JH, The effect of acetazolamide on breath holding at high altitude, Postgrad Med J 1987, 63; p. 189-190

Zandbergen J, Strahm M, Pols H, Griez EJ, Breath-holding in panic disorder, Compar Psychiatry 1992 Jan-Feb; 33(1): p. 47-51.

Asmundson GJ & Stein MB, Triggering the false suffocation alarm in panic disorder patients by using a voluntary breath-holding procedure, Am J Psychiatry 1994 Feb; 151(2): p. 264-266.

Taskar V, Clayton N, Atkins M, Shaheen Z, Stone P, Woodcock A, Breath-holding time in normal subjects, snorers, and sleep apnea patients, Chest 1995 Apr; 107(4): p. 959-962.

McNally RJ & Eke M, Anxiety sensitivity, suffocation fear, and breath-holding duration as predictors of response to carbon dioxide challenge, J Abnorm Psychol 1996 Feb; 105(1): p. 146-149.

Sasse SA, Berry RB, Nguyen TK, Light RW, Mahutte CK, Arterial Blood Gas Changes During Breath-holding From Functional Residual Capacity, Chest 1996, 110; p.958-964.

Flume PA, Eldridge FL, Edwards LJ, Mattison LE, Relief of the 'air hunger' of breathholding. A role for pulmonary stretch receptors, Respir Physiol 1996 Mar; 103(3): p. 221-232.

Marks B, Mitchell DG, Simelaro JP, Breath-holding in healthy and pulmonary-compromised populations: effects of hyperventilation and oxygen inspiration, J Magn Reson Imaging 1997 May-Jun; 7(3): p. 595-597.

Joshi LN, Joshi VD, Effect of forced breathing on ventilatory functions of the lung, J Postgrad Med. 1998 Jul-Sep; 44(3): p.67-69.

Morooka H, Wakasugi Y, Shimamoto H, Shibata O, Sumikawa K, Hyperbaric Nitrogen Prolongs Breath-Holding Time in Humans, Anesth Analg 2000; 91: p.749 –751.

Bosco G, Ionadi A, Data RG, Mortola JP, Voluntary breath-holding in the morning and in the evening Clinical Science (2004) 106, p. 347–352

Mitrouska I, Tsoumakidou M, Prinianakis G, Milic-Emili J, Siafakas NM, Effect of voluntary respiratory efforts on breath-holding time, Respiratory Physiology Neurobiology 2007, 157; p. 290–294.

Andersson JPA, Schagatay E, Repeated apneas do not affect the hypercapnic ventilatory response in the short term, Eur J Appl Physiol 2009, 105: p.569–574.

1.4 How and why the morning CP is a crucial health test

Either you already measured your CP many times or not, in both cases you are probably wondering which CP number is the most important for the Buteyko breathing method. This question is very important since the answer and attitude shape the strategy and chosen activities.

Some Buteyko breathing practitioners greatly emphasize the importance of many breathing sessions and an ability to achieve very large CP numbers during the day. These are great things. However, it is even more important to maintain the same level of health during and after sleep.

Advanced Buteyko Breathing Exercises

What are the possible problems and dangers of sleep? During the night we do not control our breathing. For most people, as was discussed before, breathing is heaviest between about 4 and 7 am. The CP is lowest during these early morning hours. Meanwhile, the main damage to the body with resetting of the breathing center corresponds to the minimum daily CP. Many positive changes due to higher daily CPs could be eliminated during sleep because of hyperventilation. The rate of overall weekly progress is reduced. The student has to start over each morning almost from the beginning.

Conclusion: **Severely sick people are most likely to die during early morning hours (4-7 am), when our breathing is heaviest and body oxygenation lowest. This fact was found for heart disease, stroke, COPD, asthma, epilepsy and many other conditions.**

Imagine, for example, what happens when the morning CP is below 10 or 20 s.

If you have bronchial asthma and acutely hyperventilate during early morning hours (as most asthmatics do), oxygenation of the body is critically low, airways become more irritated, and more inflammation is produced. Your body will try to repair airways during the day, when the CP is higher. But if you hyperventilate every morning, or even every other morning, healing will never take place. There is simply not enough time to heal since damage is systematically repeated. It is the same as scratching a wound every day until it bleeds and hoping that it will go away one day.

If you have a congenital heart disease or other abnormalities in the heart muscle, the situation is the same. You will produce considerable damage to your heart, once your CP becomes less than 10 seconds. Later you may have the best breathing exercises, a perfect diet, and many other great things, but if you hyperventilate every morning, there is no health system that can help you.

If you have cancer, your tumor will grow and even metastasize during early morning hours. Later, you can have the best diet, supplements, physical exercise, and many other wonderful things which can reduce your tumor. But if your tumor grows by about 2 mm during 2-3 hours in the morning and shrinks by 1 mm during the remaining part of the day, what would be the total effect in 1-2 months?

To find out the degree of this problem, every night, just before going to sleep, the student should measure, if there are no contra-indications, the evening CP. It will tell about the progress achieved during that particular day. Then you need to compare this number with your morning CP.

The morning CP is not just a test. It also provides us with energy and reminds us about our commitment to breathe less.

After several days of measurements, there are many numbers - daily, evening and morning CPs. Then the goal is to find out the emerging pattern related to personal circadian CP changes. Is the morning CP much smaller than the previous evening CP? By how much? Some people have relatively short sleep (e.g., about 6 hours) even when their CPs are about 10 s or less. Usually these people do not have problems with morning CP. It is nearly the same as their evening CP values.

Practice shows that over 50% of modern students have a large CP drop (at least twice) during the night sleep. For some of these people the drop is even more drastic. Only a small proportion of people (about 5-10%) have almost no difference (e.g., 1-2 s) between the evening and morning CP values.

Practicing breathing exercises and many other common sense activities gradually restores the CO_2 level back to the usual daily values. During the next night the pattern is repeated again: good daily values with about 30-70% morning CP drop.

Would the morning CP, after weeks of practice, improve, if breathing exercises and common sense activities are practiced? Practice of Buteyko breathing method practitioners shows that

Advanced Buteyko Breathing Exercises

usually it will, but low morning CP would be the greatest factor impeding the general CP progress and health restoration. It would make sense, therefore, to address the problem directly. However, the first step is to find out the degree of the problem. Hence, it is important to measure and record your morning CP.

Practicing reduced breathing, when going to sleep, helps you to remember about doing the morning CP test. In addition, it helps you to solve the problem how to fall asleep fast.

Chapter 2. Diaphragmatic breathing

2.1 Why do we need diaphragmatic breathing?

The diaphragm, in normal health, does over 75% of the work of breathing at rest (Ganong, 1995; Castro, 2000). Most modern people, as it is easy to observe, have predominantly chest breathing. Does chest breathing interfere with the health of humans and the normal functioning of the diaphragm?

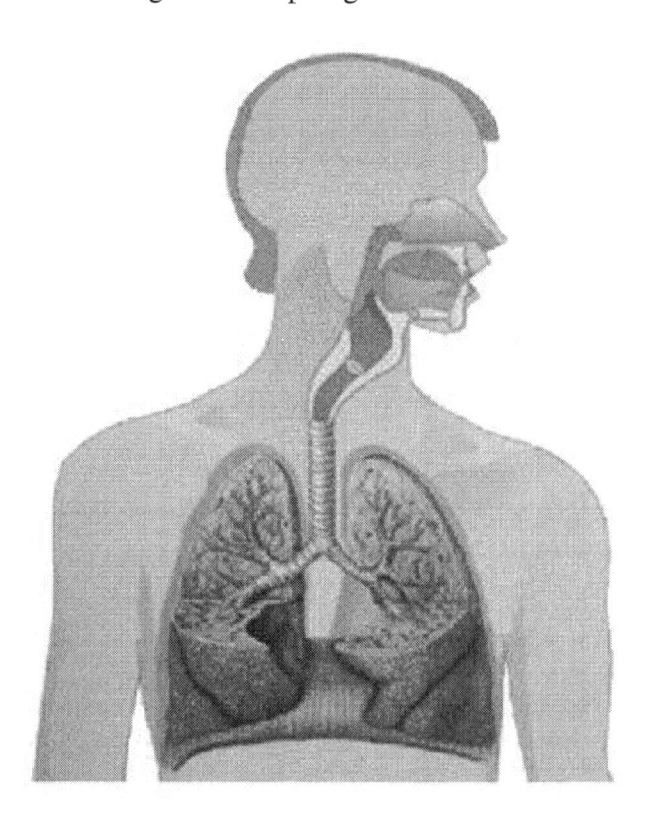

1. Yes. We need diaphragmatic breathing 24/7 to regulate *efficient* **O2 delivery and (partial) CO2 elimination.** (Note that, while the majority of modern people believe in the deep breathing myth and the poisonous nature of CO2, medical science has found dozens of benefits of CO2 in the human body.)

Advanced Buteyko Breathing Exercises

Respiratory Physiology, by John West, documents that the upper 7% of the lung delivers 4 ml of oxygen per minute, while the lower 13% of the lung brings in 60 ml of oxygen every minute (West, 2000). Therefore, lower parts of the lungs are about 7 times more productive in oxygen transport. While normal breathing at rest has a small tidal volume (only about 500 ml for a 70-kg person), it provides hemoglobin in the arterial blood with up to 98-99% O2 saturation due to the leading role of the diaphragm in the respiratory process.

In contrast, chest breathing is usually larger and deeper (up to 12-18 L/min for minute ventilation, 700-900 mL for tidal volume, and 18-25 breaths/minute in mild forms of heart disease, diabetes, asthma and so forth). But during thoracic breathing, blood oxygen levels are actually *reduced* due to inhomogeneous gas exchange: lower parts of the lungs do not get fresh air supply during chest breathing. In certain cases, this pathology (chest breathing) can greatly contribute to or even lead to pneumoperitoneum, more mucus of phlegm, emphysema, chronic respiratory fatigue, severe asthma, bronchitis, cystic fibrosis, heart disease, diabetes, cancer tumor growth, and other pathologies. (For mucus, see this link – how to get rid of phlegm.)

2. We need diaphragmatic breathing 24/7 to perform lymphatic drainage of the lymph nodes from the visceral organs. The diaphragm is a lymphatic pump, since about 60% of all lymph nodes in the human body are located just under the diaphragm. Dr. Shields, in his study, "Lymph, lymph glands, and homeostasis" (Shields, 1992), reported that diaphragmatic breathing stimulates the cleansing of the lymph nodes by creating a negative pressure pulling the lymph through the lymphatic system. This increases the rate of toxic elimination by about 15 times, as this clinical study reports.

Chest breathing at rest causes lymphatic stagnation in the stomach, pancreas, spleen, liver, kidneys, large and small colon, and other organs. Hence, effective lymphatic drainage is also among the benefits of diaphragmatic breathing.

When we switch to thoracic breathing (as during unnoticeable hyperventilation), this function of the diaphragm is taken over by the chest muscles. The resulting hypocapnia constricts bronchi and bronchioles, leading to a tenser and higher pitched voice. This effect is especially noticeable during singing, so it is not a surprise that singing teachers encourage diaphragmatic breathing in their students.

References

Shields JW, MD, Lymph, lymph glands, and homeostasis, Lymphology, Dec. 1992, 25, 4: 147.

West JB. Respiratory physiology: the essentials. 6th ed. Philadelphia: Lippincott, Williams and Wilkins; 2000.

2.2 How to test your own breathing technique

How can you check your predominant automatic breathing technique? Do you usually breathe using the belly and diaphragm or chest at rest?

Self-test. Put one hand on your stomach (or abdomen) and the other one on your upper chest (see the picture on the right). Relax completely so that your breathing dynamic has little changes. (We want to know more about your usual unconscious breathing.) Pay attention to your breathing for about 20-30 seconds. Take 2-3 very slow but deep breaths to feel your breathing in more detail.

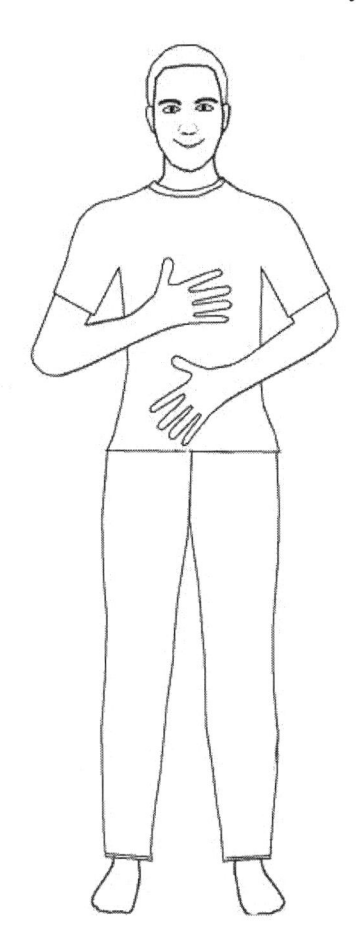

Now you know about your usual breathing technique. In order to be certain, you can ask other people to observe how you breathe when you do not pay attention to your breathing (e.g., during sleep, while reading, studying, etc.).

2.3 Causes of diaphragm dysfunction and chest breathing in modern people

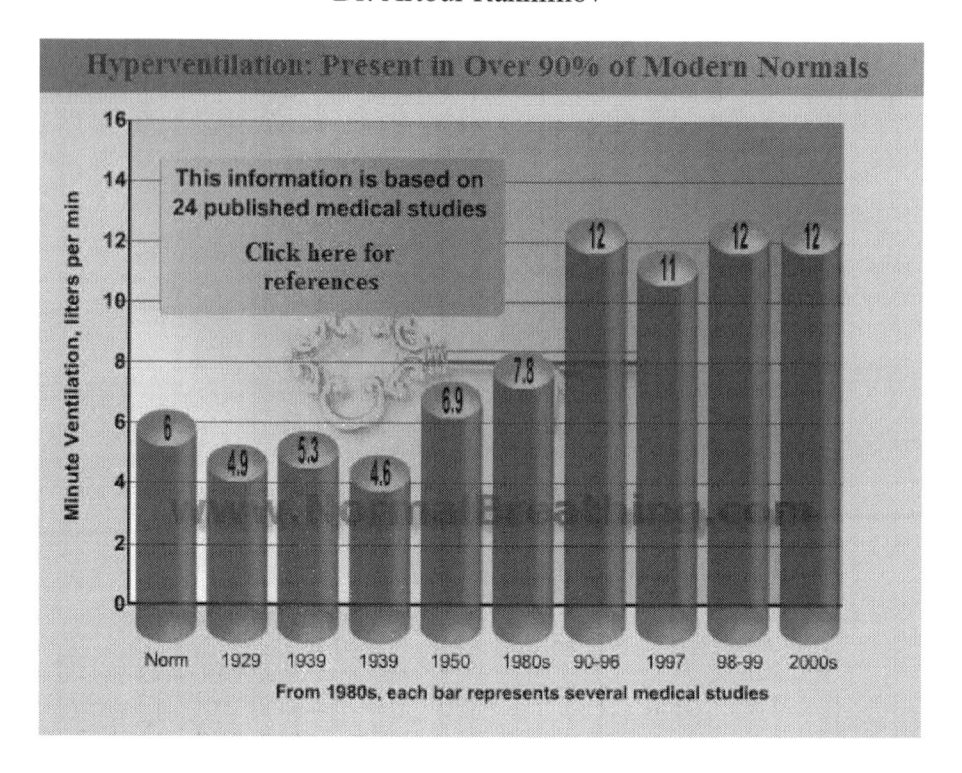

Hyperventilation: Present in Over 90% of Modern Normals

[Bar chart showing Minute Ventilation (liters per min) across years:
- Norm: 6
- 1929: 4.9
- 1939: 5.3
- 1939: 4.6
- 1950: 6.9
- 1980s: 7.8
- 90-96: 12
- 1997: 11
- 98-99: 12
- 2000s: 12

This information is based on 24 published medical studies. Click here for references.

From 1980s, each bar represents several medical studies]

Modern ordinary people breathe nearly 3 times more air than people living during first decades of the 20th century. Hyperventilation is the main, and generally the only, cause of chest breathing in modern people and their inability to enjoy the diaphragmatic breathing benefits. Let us consider why.

Alveolar hypocapnia (low CO2 in the lungs) leads to hypoxia in body cells (low body oxygenation), including the muscle cells of the diaphragm. As a result, the diaphragm gets into a state of spasm. If breathing gets slower or closer to the norm (e.g., due to breathing retraining), the oxygen level in the diaphragm will increase and it will become again the main respiratory muscle used for breathing at rest.

The situation in sick people or those who suffer from chronic diseases, such as heart disease, diabetes, cancer, asthma, and bronchitis, is even worse. These people breathe even faster and deeper than normal subjects, usually between 12 and 18 Liters per minute. There are dozens of such studies.

You can find references for this chart and for studies on respiration parameters in normal people on the web pages of the site NormalBreathing.com.

2.4 How to restore function to the diaphragm 24/7?

You can restore constant (or automatic) diaphragmatic breathing if you have more than 30 seconds for body oxygenation 24/7. Here is a chart that provides a relationship between basal breathing (measured using the body oxygen test or Buteyko Control Pause) and typical breathing at rest.

Diaphragmatic vs. chest breathing and body O2 content

Body-Oxygen Content	Automatic breathing at rest: diaphragmatic or chest?
1-10 s	Virtually always chest
11-20 s	Chest in over 90% of people
21-30 s	Mostly chest
31-40 s	Mostly belly
over 41 s	Virtually always belly

As we see from this Table, diaphragmatic breathing becomes automatic (24/7), when the body-oxygen level (CP) is over 30 s 24/7. This means that the morning CP is also more than 30 s. It is logical then that people in the past (about 100 years ago or more) had abdominal breathing 24/7 because they had more than 40 s for the body-oxygen test.

This chart also agrees with observations related to contemporary people. Indeed, since relatively healthy people have only about 20-

25 s CP these days, most people are chest breathers. Nearly all sick people are chest breathers as well.

Therefore, in order to achieve diaphragmatic breathing, you need to get more than 30 s for brain and body oxygenation 24/7.

This is the long-term goal. If we consider more immediate goals (how to learn and have diaphragmatic breathing during breathing exercises), the situation depends on various factors. The age of the person is another important factor. For younger people, in their 20's or 30's, it is much easier to learn diaphragmatic breathing. For teenagers, it is even easier. Finally, children naturally have automatic diaphragmatic breathing even when they have CPs as low as 5-7 seconds.

2.5 Specific techniques with diaphragmatic breathing: exercise with books

In order to achieve constant abdominal (or diaphragmatic) breathing, some people may require special breathing techniques.

Take 2-3 medium weight books or one large phone book and lie down on your back with the books on your tummy. Focus on your breathing and change the way you breathe so that:
1) you can lift the books up about 2-3 cm (1 inch) with each inhalation and then relax to exhale (the books will go down when you relax to exhale)
2) your rib cage does not expand during inhalations.

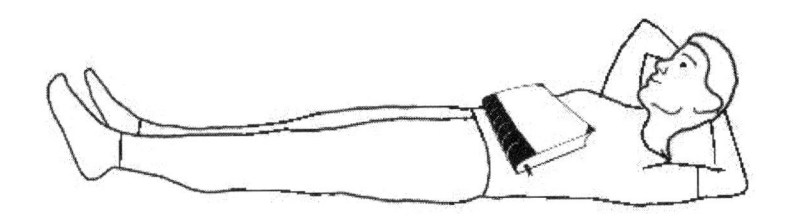

Repeat this **diaphragmatic breathing** exercise for about 3-5 minutes before your main breathing exercises to reconnect your conscious brain with the diaphragm. You can practice this exercise for some days (up to 5-7 times per day for only about 3-5 minutes each time) until you are sure that diaphragmatic breathing is the usual way to breathe during the breathing sessions.

If the diaphragm is not yet the main muscle for your automatic breathing at rest, and/or you have doubts about your ability to keep your chest muscles relaxed during breathing exercises, you can apply the following ultimate solution that blocks chest breathing.

2.6 Diaphragmatic breathing technique with belts

You can use a strong belt to restrict your rib cage and "force" the diaphragm to be the main breathing muscle using the following technique.

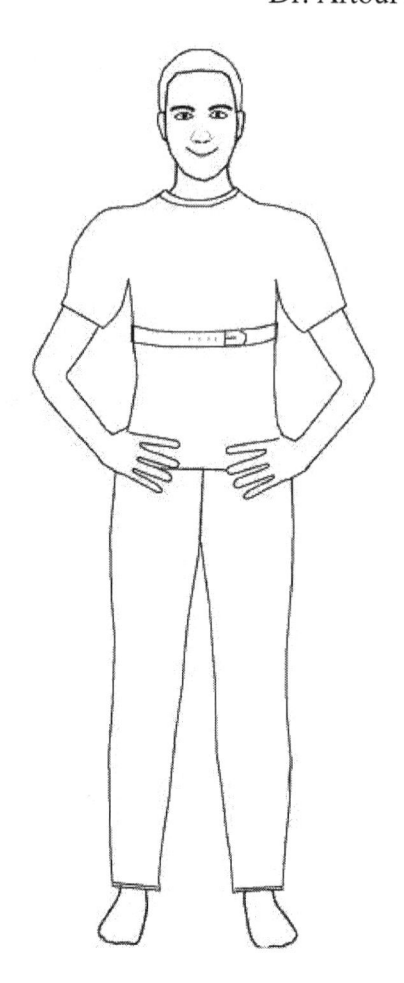

Put a belt around your lower ribs (in the middle of the trunk) and buckle it tightly so that you cannot take a deep inhalation using your rib cage or chest. Now for slow deep inhalations your body needs to use your tummy (or abdomen). Try it. While leaving the belt in place for some minutes or even hours, you can acquire diaphragmatic breathing and corresponding sensations.

There are, however, some people who will switch to upper chest breathing. This is common for elderly women who have been chest breathers for decades. In some of these women, this belt will not make any difference since they are breathing using the upper chest. Therefore, the belt does not make any difference. The solution to this problem is following: they need to use a second belt and fix it just under their armpits so that they cannot have upper chest breathing as well.

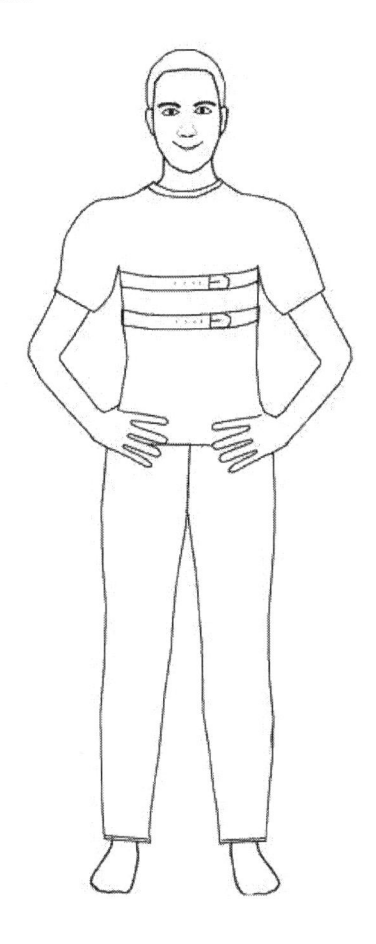

While having 2 belts, it is not possible to have any chest breathing.

For some people with persistently tense diaphragms, who in addition have problems with slouching and constipation (see <u>constipation remedies</u>), extra magnesium can be an additional assisting factor. (A lack of magnesium leads to spasm and tension in body muscles.) Elderly women and people with COPD may require up to 1-2 weeks to master abdominal breathing.

2.7 Magnesium can be a key factor for some people

The diets of modern people are low in **magnesium**, which is a known relaxant of muscles, the diaphragm included. The normal daily requirement for Mg is about 400-500 mg. Typical symptoms of magnesium deficiency include: a tendency to slouch (indicating muscular tension), predisposition to constipation (muscles of the bowel also get into a state of spasm; hence "Milk of magnesia" or magnesium oxide is a popular and safe remedy for constipation) and **tense diaphragm,** causing chest breathing 24/7. Try taking a Mg supplement (about 400-500 mg daily plus calcium to maintain a proper balance) for 3 days and monitor your symptoms and any effects on your posture, breathing mechanics and CP. (See more about this 3-day test in the manual **Major-Nutrients Guide for higher Body-Oxygen Levels**, which is freely available from NormalBreathing.com.)

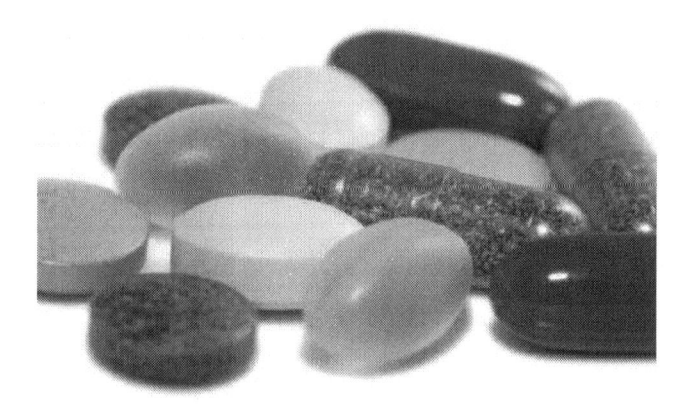

You need to restore a light and easy automatic breathing pattern or normalize your breathing in order to have abdominal breathing 24/7. What are the most effective abdominal breathing techniques? Hatha yoga and the Buteyko breathing technique are two methods to prevent chest breathing. There are even more effective ways listed below.

2.8 Advanced diaphragmatic breathing exercises for unblocking the diaphragm

While using the exercise with books (described above) and magnesium supplementation, most people with chronic diseases and an overwhelming majority of ordinary people are able to achieve success in their attempts to learn basic diaphragmatic breathing.

If you still have difficulties with diaphragmatic breathing even after using these techniques, you better start with the use of breathing devices, such as the Frolov breathing device or the Amazing DIY breathing device.

Why is it easier to learn diaphragmatic breathing with a device? The reasons are the following. When using breathing devices you can breathe more air than at rest and have large inhalations and exhalations since the devices keep your CO2. They trap the last portion of your exhaled air with the highest CO2 concentrations. In contrast, in order to practice Buteyko reduced breathing, you need to breathe less and to have shorter inhalations using the diaphragm.

If, after several days of practicing the exercise with books and using Mg supplementation, diaphragmatic breathing is still a challenge for you, then it is better for you to start breathing exercises with a breathing device. Exercises with breathing devices (for example, the Frolov device or Amazing DIY Breathing Device) are much easier since you can safely have diaphragmatic breathing with large or even nearly maximum amplitude.

Furthermore, when teaching my students during last 2 years, I found that those people who have less than 25 s for their current CPs get more benefits while using these breathing devices rather than using the Buteyko breathing exercises. Buteyko exercises become nearly equally effective when the current CP is about 30 seconds or more.

If you found that diaphragmatic breathing is easy for you, excellent, you can proceed without devices. If you get 30+ s CP in about 1-3 weeks, these weeks of practicing reduced breathing will help you in the long run.

2.9 Importance of posture for diaphragmatic breathing

It is vital for your health, abdominal breathing, good blood oxygenation, and respiratory and GI health to have a straight spine 24/7. Correct posture encourages diaphragmatic and abdominal breathing, while slouching prevents them.

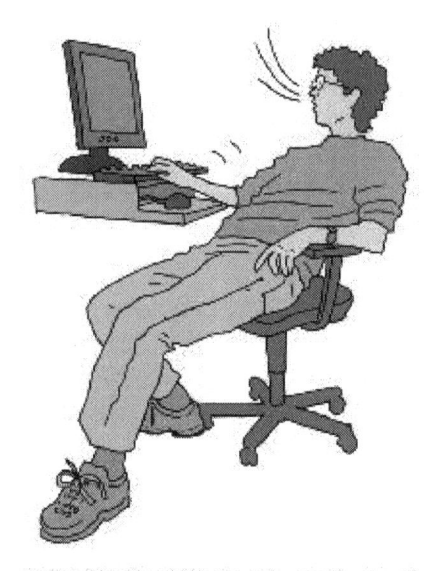

Illustration by Victor Lunn-Rockliffe

Slouching shoulders, while seemingly relaxing, leads to stress and tension in various muscles. Most of all, it causes chest breathing since the diaphragm becomes immobile. During quiet breathing at rest we need the diaphragm to do the main work of breathing (up to about 90%, as many medical textbooks suggest). Hence, slouching shoulders immediately causes chest breathing with reversal of breathing modes: up to 90% of respiratory movements will be done by the chest muscles.

Slouching shoulders make breathing deeper and faster leading to chronic hyperventilation that causes low body-oxygen content, poor body oxygen test results and ... more slouching. Why?

Relationships between body oxygen level and chances of slouching

Body-Oxygen Level	Minute Ventilation*	Chance of slouching
Less than 20 s	Over 12 L/min	Likely
20-30 s	9-12 L/min	Possible
30-40 s	6-9 L/min	Almost impossible
>40 s	<6 L/min	Virtually impossible

* Minute ventilation for a 70-kg person at rest

Clinical experience of Russian doctors shows that slouching intensifies breathing causing a lack of CO_2 in the lungs and the arterial blood. Since CO_2 is a potent vasodilator (see Vasodilation) and required for the Bohr effect, poor posture immediately reduces oxygen content in the cells. This promotes chronic diseases since they are based on tissue hypoxia. It is normal then that some people can experience chest pain, angina pain, exacerbations of digestive problems, heart palpitations and arrhythmias due to slouching. Hence, they should stop slouching shoulders.

Less than 10% of modern people have normal breathing parameters and over 40 s for the body oxygen test. It is not a surprise then that most modern people have poor posture. Slouching shoulders is a norm in public schools, universities, libraries, and other places. However, if you watch old movies and investigate old pictures and photos, you can notice that people living during first decades of the 20th century naturally had a good posture with no slouching.

Furthermore, the problem is even worse in people with chronic diseases since their heavy breathing makes muscles even more tense and oxygen deficient. As a result, generally, the sicker the person, the stronger the slouching. To stop slouching shoulders is easy with breathing retraining. At higher body-oxygen levels, correct posture becomes normal naturally.

Generally, people stop slouching completely and naturally when they get over 40 s for their morning CP. However, when a person with about 25-30 s has a poor posture, his or her breathing gets worse and the CP drops.

My suggestion is that, if you have more than 15 s for the CP test, you need to consciously correct your posture 24/7. Later, with higher CPs, it will be much easier for your body to maintain correct posture automatically.

Chapter 3. Restrictions, limits, and temporary contraindications

Normal breathing is the fundamental property of the healthy organism. Hence, breathing normalization is the natural way to deal with many pathologies or diseases of the human body. However, not all people can use the same method in their breathing normalization. While most people can apply the same exercises and techniques (including Buteyko reduced breathing exercise), there are groups of people who require individual tailoring and adjustments in their breathing retraining programs due to certain restrictions, limits, and temporary contraindications.

You should adjust your program and follow specific instructions, if you have:
- Migraine headaches, panic attacks, and heart disease (aortic aneurysms; angina pectoris; arrhythmia; atherosclerosis (plaque buildup); cardiomyopathy; ciliary arrhythmia (cardiac fibrillation); chest pain (angina pectoris); high cholesterol; chronic ischemia; congenital heart disease; congestive heart failure; coronary artery disease; endocarditis; extrasystole; heart murmurs; hypertension; hypertrophic cardiomyopathy; tachycardia; pericarditis; post-myocardial infarction; stroke)
- Presence of transplanted organs
- Pregnancy
- Brain traumas and acute bleeding injuries
- Blood clots
- Acute stages (exacerbations) of life-threatening conditions (infarct, stroke, cardiac ischemia, severe asthma attack, metastasizing cancer, septic shock, multiple organ failure, near-death experience, etc.)
- Insulin-dependent diabetes (type 2 diabetes)
- Loss of CO2 sensitivity
- Low weight (underweight)
- Been using many types of prescribed medical drugs.

Warning: Consult your family physician or GP about the use of these breathing exercises for your specific health problems. Slower breathing and increased body oxygenation increase the effects of many types of medical drugs and can cause undesirable symptoms.

3.1 Heart disease, migraine headaches, and panic attacks

These restrictions and conditions are for people with:
Heart disease (aortic aneurysms; angina pectoris; arrhythmia; atherosclerosis (plaque buildup); cardiomyopathy; ciliary arrhythmia (cardiac fibrillation); chest pain (angina pectoris); high cholesterol; chronic ischemia; congenital heart disease; congestive heart failure; coronary artery disease; endocarditis; extrasystole; heart murmurs; hypertension; hypertrophic cardiomyopathy; pericarditis; post-myocardial infarction; stroke; tachycardia)
Migraine headaches and panic attacks.

Depending on the severity and type of the condition and some other personal factors, many of these patients can worsen their health state if they try intensive breathing sessions accompanied by quick CO_2 increases. Predisposed patients can even develop higher blood pressure, panic attacks, and migraine headaches.

Even a CP measurement can trigger negative cardiovascular changes in some heart patients. Note that other groups of people can do breath holds without any negative effects, but the blood vessels of some heart patients can constrict due to too quick changes in blood gas composition. This effect was known to Dr. K. Buteyko, who described it in his medical publication in the 1960's.

Advanced Buteyko Breathing Exercises

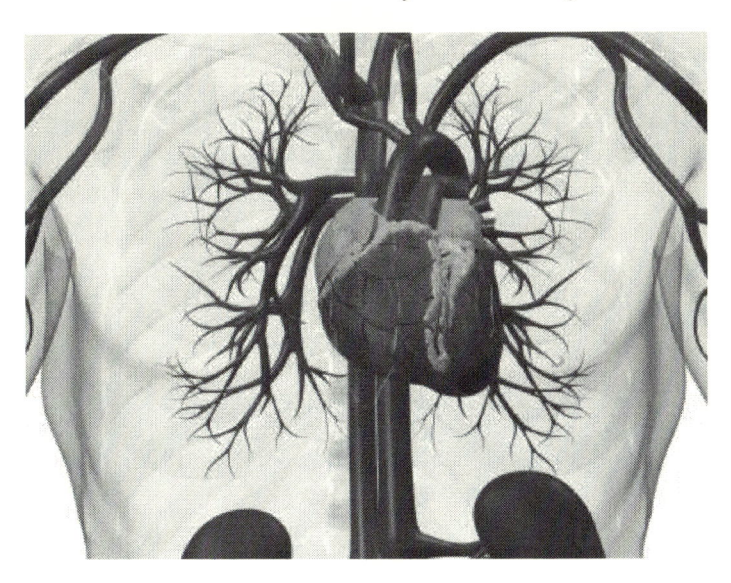

Many of these patients (with heart disease, migraine headaches, or panic attacks) can practice the main breathing exercises, including the reduced breathing developed by Dr. Buteyko. However, in order to be safe, it is better for these people to start with lighter forms of breathing exercises.

When practicing Buteyko breathing exercises, various pauses and reduced breathing, follow these instructions.

If you feel uncomfortable/overstressed after doing the CP test and any other pauses (including maximum and extended pauses) and your heart rate gets higher (3-5 min after the test), do not do any breath holds. It is a known effect that some groups of people get an abnormal cardiovascular response with constriction of the blood vessels, as a reaction to sudden and sharp changes in arterial CO_2. Breathing sessions and exercises should lead to a higher CP, a lower heart rate and an improved feeling of well-being. Hence, you need to adjust your breathing exercises to your current (temporary) state by avoiding uncomfortable pauses and focusing on reduced breathing.

Your goal for the Buteyko breathing exercises is to reduce your heart rate after the session. Start with the relaxation of the diaphragm exercise that does not create any sensation of air hunger. (This exercise is explained below.) Practice this exercise for several days and then try the CP test again. Later you can proceed to more demanding exercises and start practicing reduced breathing without any pauses (as it is described on the web page Learn Buteyko reduced breathing).

When your breathing, after some days/weeks of practice becomes lighter, the ability to do pauses is improved (you can safely do, for example, the CP measurement) and they are safe and useful to do. For example, with over 20 s CP such people are comfortable doing the CPs and even practicing the reduced breathing immediately after the CP without any unpleasant sensations. Then you can practice a regular Buteyko breathing exercise session.

When such students (panic attacks, heart disease, or migraine headaches) get over 30 s CP, no restrictions are usually necessary, extended and maximum pauses are safe, and these students can join the main group in further breathing normalization.

Keep in mind, that at any stage, it is important that you feel better after the breathing sessions and your heart rate should become lower either immediately after the breathing session or 5-10 minutes later.

Important note for patients with high blood pressure. Within 3-4 days after starting breathing retraining, people with hypertension experience a better quality of life (more energy, better concentration, alertness, sleep and digestion). However, they often experience a very light increase in blood pressure (about 10-15 mm Hg) during the first 5-7 days of breathing retraining. During the following 2-6 weeks their blood pressure gets back to normal. It is very important for them to practice regularly.

When practicing the relaxation of the diaphragm (a special Buteyko breathing exercise for patients with high blood pressure), these people should not try to create any air hunger or sensation of shortage of air.

3.2 Presence of transplanted organs

You should not have more than 30 s for your CP (preferably less than 27 s) at any time of the day to prevent rejection of the transplanted organs. When the CP gets more than 30 s (it corresponds to transition to the next health zone according to the Buteyko Table of Health Zones), the immune system can become more sensitive to foreign tissues and cells and can launch an attack on these tissues in an attempt to repair them.

However, depending on differences in DNAs or a matching of the transplanted organ (transplant compatibility), some students can safely achieve 30, 40 s or even higher CPs.

3.3 Breathing exercises during pregnancy

The main danger during pregnancy is a spontaneous abortion that can happen due to a cleansing reaction caused by a very fast progress in body-oxygen test results due to breathing retraining.

Imagine a pregnant woman who starts with about 10-12 s CP. Note that hyperventilation, hypocapnia, reduced perfusion, hypoxemia, headaches, cramps, and many other effects of hyperventilation (hypertension, asthma, poor blood sugar control, anxiety, dry cough, and many other effects) are common in pregnant females these days. Then assume that she achieves 35-40 s for the body-oxygen test in 4-6 days due to intensive breathing retraining.

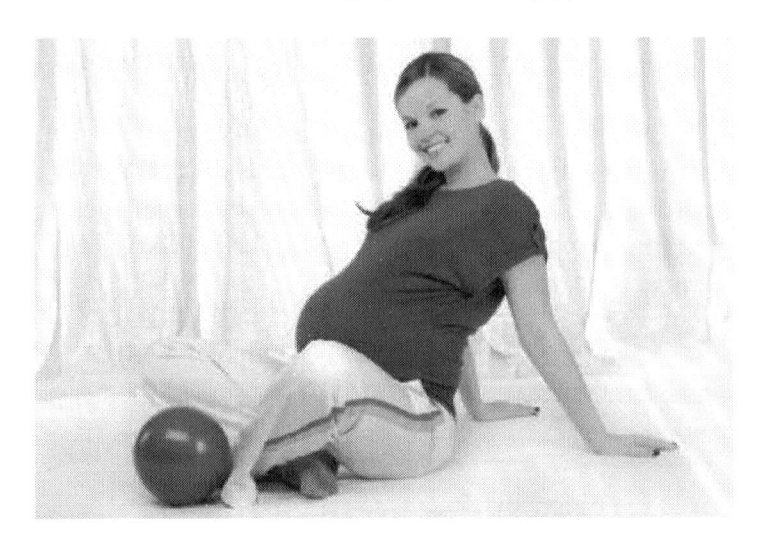

Her automatic or unconscious breathing pattern becomes much slower and lighter. Her body oxygenation gets much higher. The immune system becomes highly sensitive to abnormal tissues and is able to reject transplanted organs, as we considered above. Similarly, the immune system at higher CPs can easily reject an embryo at the state when it is not yet attached to the womb of the mother (the first trimester of the pregnancy), as Buteyko breathing doctors discovered during the 1960's. The chances of spontaneous abortion are much higher, if the growing embryo accumulated medical drugs or if the mother has been taking medication before and immediately after getting pregnant.

In order to prevent this scenario, the pregnant woman should have a defensive program of breathing retraining based on prevention of large CP fluctuations or CP losses (episodes of hyperventilation) due to overeating, mouth breathing, supine sleep, poor posture, morning hyperventilation, etc. The rate of the CP progress while learning the Buteyko technique or using breathing devices (e.g., the Frolov device or DIY breathing device) should be limited:
- for women who used medical drugs for a long time or were exposed to toxic chemicals by 2 s in one week;
- for other pregnant women by 3 s in one week.

3.4 Brain traumas and acute bleeding injuries

Hyperventilation is a normal and useful reaction to bleeding injuries. Reduced CO2 content in the blood decreases the blood flow to vital organs and other tissues of the human body. This prevents excessive blood losses and can save one's life. Emergency professionals even coined a term "permissive hyperventilation" that is used for people with, for example, brain trauma.

Therefore, it is beneficial, and sometimes life-saving, to hyperventilate when having acute injuries with bleeding. You should not try to reduce your automatic breathing in such conditions.

Later, when bleeding has ceased, it is possible to follow the common program, if there are no other restrictions.

3.5 Blood clots

Reduced breathing dilates the arteries and arterioles and makes the blood thinner so that existing blood clots could get loose and travel via the blood. The released clot may block the blood flow through the artery leading to the brain or heart muscle and cause death.

Hence, a person with a blood clot will benefit from avoiding maximum pauses, extended pauses, control pauses and other breath holds that cause sudden dilation of arteries and arterioles. Breathing exercises (Buteyko technique, Frolov device, and so forth) should be short and the weekly CP (control pause of body oxygen level) growth should be limited to 1-2 seconds only. It is better to focus on defensive measures in relation to breathing retraining (prevention of CP drops due to sleep, mouth breathing, slouching, overheating, and so on). These defensive activities prevent periods of hyperventilation that make the blood thicker and the clot larger.

Other beneficial lifestyle changes are physical exercise with strictly nose breathing and a good diet. In particular, a raw vegetarian diet and natural enzymes or supplements can be great assisting factors to dissolve the blood clot naturally.

Later, when the clot is dissolved or removed, the person can follow the common program of breathing retraining adjusted to their new health state. Depending on diet and CP fluctuations, the natural process of blood clot dissolving takes place between 20 and 35 seconds. The same CP numbers are necessary to prevent formation of blood clots.

3.6 Acute stages (exacerbations) and life-threatening conditions

This section relates to people with infarct, stroke, cardiac ischemia, severe asthma attack, metastasizing cancer, septic shock, multiple organ failure, near-death experience, and other very serious conditions.

Modern EM (Emergency Medicine) professionals developed many successful and useful methods and techniques for people in critical care and life-threatening states. Breathing retraining cannot replace these techniques (CPR, breathing pure oxygen, etc.) when people are unconscious or unable to have a good control of their actions due to their very poor health state.

Breathing exercises cannot stop quickly progressing metastasizing cancer (stages 3 and 4).

Later, when the person is in a stable state, these people can follow the Buteyko method program of breathing retraining adjusted to their new health state.

3.7 Loss of CO2 sensitivity

Loss of CO2 sensitivity is a specific topic that can be very important for some students. Unfortunately, most Western Buteyko trainers and practitioners do not have any information or even tests and practical approaches to solve this problem. It is discussed in detail in Oxygen Remedy. Some guidelines are also provided in this book.

This problem is caused by a too large alveolar CO2 increase and takes place only in a small number of people who are genetically predisposed to heart disease, suffer from allergies, inflammation, low body weight, overheating, a lack of Ca and arginine in their diet, and/or lack of deep stages of sleep. It is a combination of factors that leads to loss of CO2 sensitivity.

Loss of CO2 sensitivity causes vasoconstriction and reduced blood flow to vital organs. The effect can cause headaches and drastically reduce the well-being of a person.

Loss of CO2 sensitivity is manifested in the dys-regulation of breathing and a sudden increase in the resting pulse, generally up to 90 beats per minute or more. The effect can last for hours, weeks, or months depending on the lifestyle and changes made.

Practical note
You may suspect that you have this problem, only if your heart rate is about 20 or beats higher than your usual numbers. For example, your usual pulse at rest while sitting is about 70 beats/min. If later your heart rate constantly stays above 90 beats per minute, you may have this challenge with lost CO2 sensitivity.

3.8 Breathing exercises for underweight (or low weight) people

The most natural way how to gain weight fast is to improve the digestive system, the liver function, and the appetite (or hunger) naturally by increasing the body-oxygen levels. When a person is underweight and struggles with weight gain, he or she always has low body oxygenation, generally less than 20 seconds for the body-oxygen test. This means chest breathing 24/7 (which drastically reduces blood oxygenation), possible mouth breathing (especially at night), and chronic overbreathing or breathing more than the norm. These abnormalities cause poor perfusion of all organs, a lack of hunger, low levels of energy, a horrible quality of sleep and many other problems. This how to gain weight approach suggests removing the cause of all these problems: too fast and too deep chest breathing.

Note that apart from low body oxygenation, hyperventilation or fast and deep breathing can also increase blood glucose levels, and while having low energy levels due to tissue hypoxia, such underweight people are not hungry and that causes problems with how to gain weight. This can be easily reversed with correct breathing exercises.

It is a very common effect that when underweight or too slim people start practicing the Buteyko breathing exercises, their blood glucose level drops since the body is "inviting" new calories to be used for weight gain with the goal to get your body weight closer to the norm. Therefore, **these people may require a snack immediately after breathing exercises** especially if they start to feel cold and hungry. People with very low weight can eat more, but only until their hunger disappears.

3.9 Breathing exercises and prescribed medical drugs

Many types of medical drugs become more potent with higher CPs. Most doctors do not know this effect and they adjust dosages of medical drugs arbitrary. There are many guidelines related to dosages. However, since these guidelines do not take into account breathing patterns of patients, many people get too much medication, and some too little. In addition, most doctors prescribe medication for fixed periods of time. Soviet Buteyko doctors realized that the dosages of nearly all types of medical drugs should be adjusted to the current CP of a patient.

For example, people with severe **hypertension** require large dosages of antihypertensives (medications to lower blood pressure). This is logical since such people have only about 8-12 s (or less) for their CPs. However, when the same person with hypertension increases his or her CP up to about 15 seconds, they may need about 2-3 times less medication. If they continue to use the same dose, they can get a too low blood pressure, and this can cause other serious symptoms and problems. With over 20 s for the morning CP, most such people have a normal blood pressure without drugs. Therefore, any medication that lowers their blood pressure can become dangerous.

A similar situation was discovered by Soviet Buteyko doctors in relation to **diabetics** who take insulin or other types of medication that lowers the blood glucose levels. However, people with diabetes still require insulin even when they have 25 s for the morning CP. This is because the body starts to produce more insulin at higher CPs, and this insulin becomes more effective. Insulin becomes unnecessary when a person has about 35 s for the morning CP with less than 70 beats per minute for pulse at rest. This was the conclusion reported by Dr. Buteyko and Dr. Angelina Nikolaevna Samotesova, Chief Endocrinologist of the Krasnoyarsk region during the 2nd Conference of Soviet Buteyko breathing doctors in 1991. Note that an insulin overdose is potentially very dangerous. Fortunately, nearly all contemporary diabetics use glucometers (devices to measure glucose levels in the blood) in order to define the next dose of medication to lower blood glucose.

People with **hypothyroidism** are often prescribed thyroxine. The effect of this hormone is also CP-related. For example, a person with this condition can increase the CP from 10 up to 20 s. At this higher CP level (20 s), the body starts to produce its own thyroxine. The same dosage of thyroid medication can cause too high blood levels of thyroxine causing heart palpitations and other adverse symptoms. With over 35 s for the morning CP, there is no need for this thyroid medication.

Therefore, if you take any type of medication, it is good to know and discuss these effects with your health care provider. Most importantly, you need to pay close attention to your symptoms and report them to your health care provider so that he or she can adjust or change your medication.

Chapter 4. Buteyko exercises for beginners

4.1 Preliminary requirements for learning Buteyko breathing exercises

A quiet place to focus one's attention

A session requires about 15 min (or from about 12 up to 40 minutes) of concentrated work without disturbances and interruptions. Being totally concentrated is important during the initial stages of learning. Later, after many hours of practice, breathing exercises can be done while driving a car, watching TV, reading, etc.

Silence (no speaking)

You should be silent and the mouth should be closed during the whole session. If it is necessary to speak, for whatever urgent reasons, air hunger is lost and later you should hold your breath to restore a light level of air hunger (more about this desire or air hunger is below).

Empty stomach

The exercises are done on an empty stomach (water is OK) since reduced breathing and larger aCO_2 concentrations provide more blood and oxygen for the GI system intensifying peristalsis. Many modern people have an inflammation in the stomach they are unaware of, as recent western studies revealed. This inflammation can get worse due to the intensification of peristalsis in the stomach and duodenum, if food is present there. (Imagine what could happen if somebody starts to rub vigorously skin areas which are already inflamed.) Having water in the stomach does not cause this problem.

Warning. If you are hungry and have problems with blood glucose control, in many situations breathing exercises or reduced breathing will not prevent a further blood sugar drop and, in certain cases, can even intensify hypoglycemia. If this is the case for you, make sure that you are not hungry. You should not have a low or very low blood glucose level during the breathing session.

Warning. If you suffer from diabetes and use insulin, the reduced breathing will increase your sensitivity to insulin. This will make your blood sugar level lower than usual. You may suffer from hypoglycemic shock, which is much more dangerous than high blood sugar. Hypoglycemic shock, which often happens after an insulin overdose as well, can be fatal. Buteyko breathing exercises lead to reduced requirements in insulin.

Hydration (water)

The acidification of blood due to an increased CO_2 content caused by reduced breathing triggers biological pH buffers in the blood. A part of this process is the redistribution of ions in various compartments of the body (intracellular fluid, extra-cellular fluid, blood plasma, intestinal content, etc.). These processes may require additional water. Hence, drink if you get thirsty at any stage.

Clean and fresh air

The place for exercises should have clean and fresh air so that the student can have a cold and moist nose, as naturally happens outdoors. Backyards of houses, balconies or parks are great places, provided that it is not too cold or warm and there is no draught and no direct sunlight. Kitchens with open windows usually provide good conditions. Having long or old and dusty curtains, carpets, books in the room makes air stale and dusty, and many students cannot reduce their breathing in such conditions. Those people who are allergic or sensitive to dust mites, mold, proteins from cats and dogs, and other air-born substances should find a trigger-free place where no even mild allergic reaction is possible. Air ionizers can greatly improve the indoor air quality.

Thermoregulation

Find a comfortable place without draught, but relatively cool. You may feel warm or even hot during the exercises. Therefore, be ready for that to happen and take steps to restore your thermal comfort: take some clothes off to normalize your heat exchange. If a place is too warm, it is often impossible to reduce breathing and increase the CP there.

If your current CP is less than 20 s, you should be on a slighter warm side. Hence, keep yourself comfortably warm when in a poor health state or with a low CP.

If your CP is above 20 s and you have normal well-being (no signs of a cold, flu, or infection, etc.), keep yourself moderately cool. This factor will help you with your further CP growth and health restoration.

If the surrounding temperature is 25 degrees C or more, it is impossible to reduce breathing (you may try to exercise in a wet T-shirt).

Posture during the breathing session

Severely sick students with low initial CPs (less than 10 s) can do breathing exercises while lying, half-lying or sitting in a comfortable armchair with their backs supported. It is more important for them to have proper relaxation, since physical exertion can significantly intensify their breathing.

When the CP is above 10 s, it is suggested to practice while sitting on the edge of a solid chair (on half of a chair) without using the back support. You can have your elbows and arms either on the table or on your knees. **The spine should be straight and erect.** That is another crucial parameter for breathing normalization.

Warning. *If you suffer from back pain now, you can lean on the back of a chair or choose some other posture that is comfortable for you and will make relaxation possible. Your back pain may relate to calcium metabolism (and then normalization of breathing will help* *you to solve this problem) or it may relate to a displaced vertebra or a pinched nerve in your spine (and then a visit to an experienced chiropractor can solve this problem; Dr. Buteyko and his wife Ludmila learned chiropractic techniques since breathing normalization alone cannot help in all cases).*

How to check one's posture? There is a simple test. You only need any flat vertical surface (e.g., a wall or door).

The "wall test" for correct posture

Go to any flat wall (or door) and attach the back part of your whole body to this wall so that you can touch the wall with following 6 points at the same time:
- both back sides of your shoes; 2 points
- your lowest vertebra (tail bone); 1 point
- both your shoulder blades; 2 points
- the back of your head. 1 point

Some people find that they are looking too high (probably they have a habit to look down at the ground in front of them). Hence, you may feel that you are looking too high. The position of your head is not as crucial as the position of your spine. It is important that this test helps to restore the normal position of the spine so that breathing retraining is possible.

Now you can sit down on the edge of a chair while keeping the spine straight. This sitting posture is the most common posture used for those Buteyko breathing exercises that are done at rest. One can sit on a low chair with crossed legs, so that the thighs are inclined towards the floor. Then light diaphragmatic breathing is also possible. People, who can relax in lotus or other similar yoga postures (e.g., "Pleasant" posture), can do so.

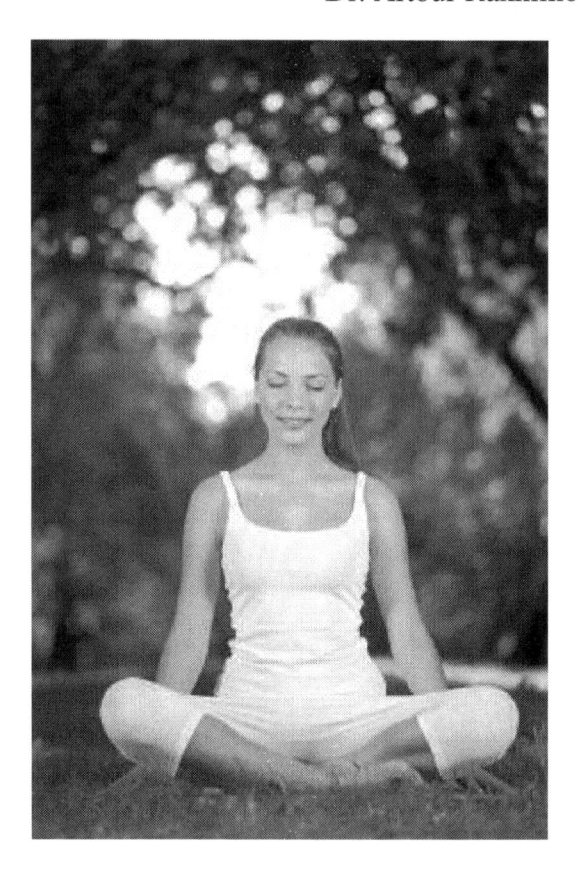

It is important for the position of the diaphragm that the thighs are either horizontal or inclined downwards when we are in the sitting position. If the thighs are inclined upwards, as when we sit on a low chair, the diaphragm is compressed by the internal organs and it loses its mobility. Diaphragmatic breathing requires a straight spine so that the diaphragm, instead of being compressed, is freely suspended and can easily be moved down and up.

4.2 The simple mechanics of normal breathing at rest or how the diaphragm works

Make your spine like a broomstick, with your shoulders, chest and belly freely hanging on this solid frame. This posture allows for shorter breaths (even during daily normal life) and the right place for various organs in the body. The reduction of unnecessary muscular

Advanced Buteyko Breathing Exercises

tension and elimination of internal pressure under the diaphragm also allows for easier breathing. This posture should be preserved for the rest of the day, but it is particularly important during the exercises. Otherwise, due to the muscular tension and stress in vital organs, the normalization of breathing during the exercises is very difficult or impossible.

Remember, when your CP gets larger and approaches 30 seconds, the posture becomes more and more important. For example, when your CP is about 15-20 s, slouching causes a 1-2 s CP decrease, while a straight spine 1-2 s more. Once you get about 25-30 s CP, a poor posture, if present, will be the factor making further health and CP progress impossible.

It is assumed that you know how to measure the CP, since the test is described on previous pages of the educational section of the website. If you are not sure about the correct procedure for the CP measurements, it is necessary to find and learn more about the CP test.

Here is a summary of 7 preliminary requirements:
- A quiet place to focus one's attention
- Silence (no speaking)
- Empty stomach
- Hydration (water)
- Clean and fresh air
- Thermoregulation
- Posture during the breathing session

4.3 Breathing patterns

Healthy people (over 40 s for the CP test or the body-oxygen test) naturally have normal diaphragmatic breathing at rest. This graph below shows the normal breathing pattern for an adult. Each cycle has a tiny inhalation (the upward straight lines), exhalation (the curved downward lines) and automatic pause (the almost horizontal lines) accompanied by the relaxation of all breathing muscles.

Normal Breathing Pattern

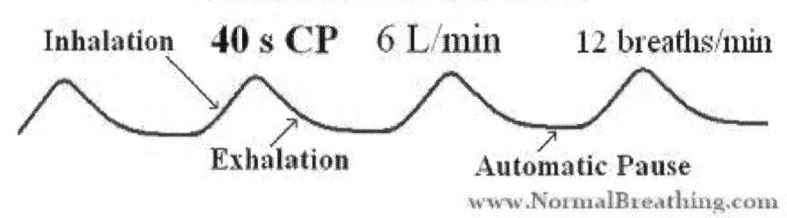

(Diagram showing breathing waveform with labels: Inhalation, Exhalation, Automatic Pause, 40 s CP, 6 L/min, 12 breaths/min)

www.NormalBreathing.com

The physiological norms for breathing at rest for an adult include:
- 6 liters per minute for minute ventilation
- 12 breaths per minute for respiratory frequency
- about 40 seconds for the CP (Control Pause).

If the CP (body-oxygen content) is about 20 s or less, as is the case with sick people, the typical breathing pattern is the following:

Breathing Pattern in the Sick

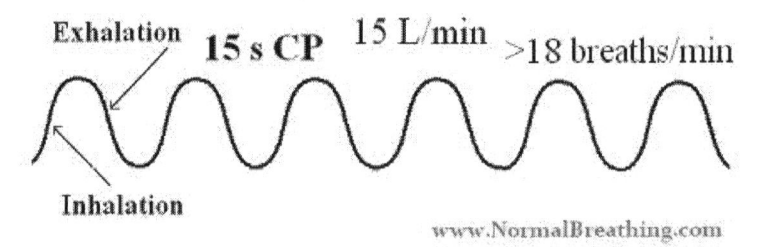

(Diagram showing breathing waveform with labels: Exhalation, Inhalation, 15 s CP, 15 L/min, >18 breaths/min)

www.NormalBreathing.com

The inhalations are bigger (deeper); breathing is faster (higher frequency); **exhalations are forceful** (not relaxed), and there is no automatic pause.

Severely sick people breathe even faster and have less than 10 s for their body oxygenation. NormalBreathing.com provides numerous studies and the exact numbers for breathing rates in people with advanced cancer, HIV-AIDS and other conditions.

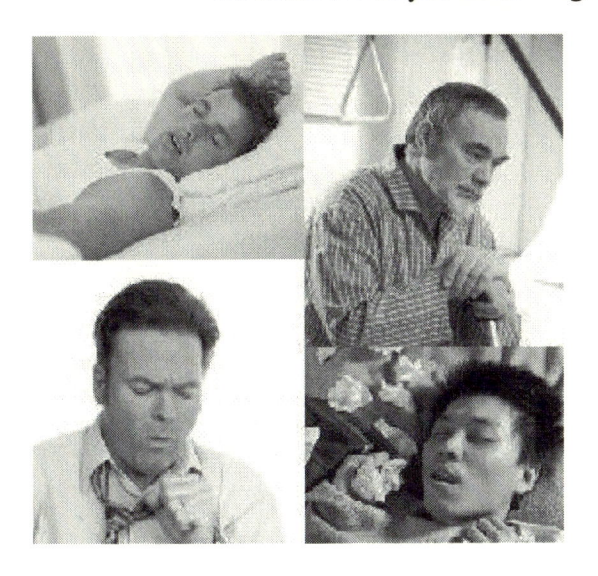

Advanced Buteyko Breathing Exercises

In order to see the general picture (and possibly your ultimate goals), here are 4 breathing patterns and their parameters.

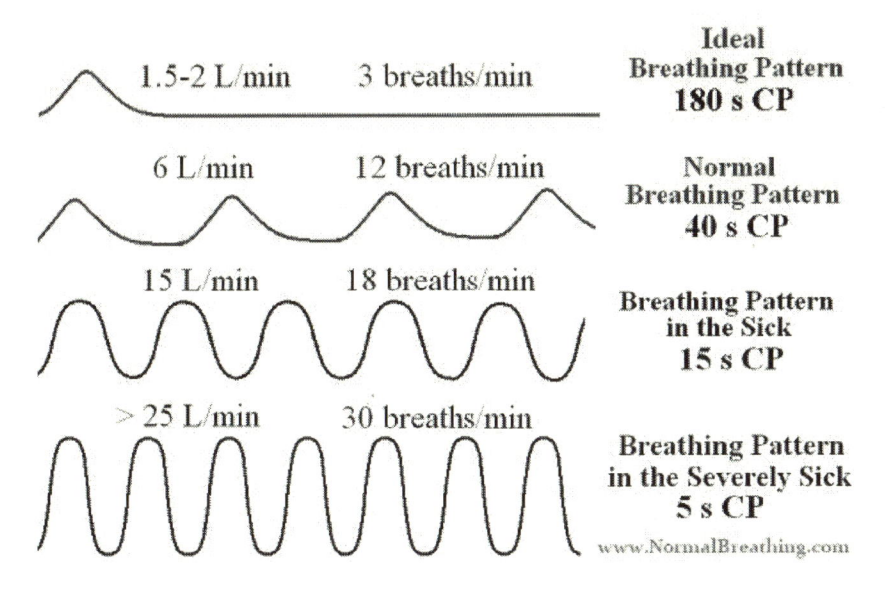

Pattern	Volume	Rate	Description
	1.5-2 L/min	3 breaths/min	**Ideal Breathing Pattern** 180 s CP
	6 L/min	12 breaths/min	**Normal Breathing Pattern** 40 s CP
	15 L/min	18 breaths/min	**Breathing Pattern in the Sick** 15 s CP
	> 25 L/min	30 breaths/min	**Breathing Pattern in the Severely Sick** 5 s CP

www.NormalBreathing.com

Warning. It is a serious mistake and a waste of time to practice normal breathing if your CP is less than 30 s. Why? People start to breathe deeply, while during normal breathing inhalations are tiny (normal breathing is invisible). Dr. Buteyko noticed this effect over

40 years ago (his quote is a few lines below). In fact, you will learn soon that reduced breathing, the main part of the Buteyko breathing exercises, is more shallow and, for sick people, more frequent.

"The breathing [retraining] should be monitored by an instructor who had learned the method himself. Our instruction of 1964 was published in Novosibirsk, 1000 issues. We still were naive and thought that after reading this correct instruction, the patient would be able to reduce breathing and then compare when it is normal. It [the instruction] included the information about normal breathing: 2 s for inhalation, 3 s for exhalation, 3 s for the pause, etc. First, he [the student] starts to breathe deeply, secondly, he immediately tries to fulfill that normal breathing. All [final] effects are the opposite, even [for] a [medical] doctor." Dr. Buteyko, Public Lecture in the Moscow State University, 1969.

4.4 Buteyko Table of Health Zones

After analyzing thousands of sick, healthy and very healthy people, Dr. Buteyko suggested the Table that I call the Buteyko Table of Health Zones.

Health state	Type of breathing	Degree	Pulse, /min	Rf, breaths /min	CO_2 in alveoli, %	AP, s	CP, s	MP, s
Super-health	Shallow	5	48	3	7.5	16	180	210
		4	50	4	7.4	12	150	190
		3	52	5	7.3	9	120	170
		2	55	6	7.1	7	100	150
		1	57	7	6.8	5	80	120
Normal	Normal	-	60	8	6.5	4	60	90
Disease	Deep	-1	65	10	6.0	3	50	75
		-2	70	12	5.5	2	40	60
		-3	75	15	5.0	-	30	50
		-4	80	20	4.5	-	20	40
		-5	90	26	4.0	-	10	20
		-6	100	30	3.5	-	5	10

Advanced Buteyko Breathing Exercises

Comments on Buteyko Table of Health Zones. Pulse – heart rate or pulse rate in 1 minute; Breathing or Respiratory frequency in one minute (number of inhalations or exhalations); % CO2 - %CO2 in alveoli of the lungs (*or arterial blood if there is no mismatch); AP - the Automatic Pause or natural delay in breathing after exhalation (*during unconscious breathing); CP - the Control Pause (body-oxygen test, breath holding time after usual exhalation and until first distress only); MP (the Maximum Pause, breath holding time after usual exhalation and as long as possible).

This discovery is patented (see the bottom of this page) and the table is based on Buteyko KP, The method of volitional elimination of deep breathing [Translation of the Small Buteyko Manual], Voskresensk, 1994.

* Note about pulse. Not all people with low CPs (less than 20 s) have a greatly increased heart rate, as is given by this table. Some categories of people with less than 20 s CP can have a resting pulse of around 60 – 70 beats per minute. However, an increased heart rate for lower CPs is the feature of, for example, heart patients and patients with severe asthma. During the 1960's, when conducting his research, and later, Buteyko and his colleagues applied the Buteyko breathing retraining program mainly for heart and asthma patients, who were mostly hospitalized with frequent deficiencies in their blood cortisol levels. This explains the increased heart rates provided by the Table.

For more information about this Table and the health effects of breathing retraining, you can find relevant pages on NormalBreathing.com.

4.5 Feeling the breath and learning how to relax

This big and deep breathing usually makes the chest muscles to do the main job of air pumping. Why? Low CO2 content makes the diaphragm tense. Coupled with slouching, it restricts diaphragmatic movements making chest breathing the typical feature of people with low CPs.

If you have been using mostly your chest muscles for breathing at rest during the last 5-10 or more years, it could take you some weeks to restore the normal diaphragmatic breathing.

The process of learning to unblock the diaphragm is divided into 4 stages:
Stage 1: Feeling the breath
Stage 2: Relaxation of the body's muscles
Stage 3: Tensing and relaxing breathing muscles
Stage 4: Relaxed diaphragmatic breathing

Stage 1: Feeling the breath

Focus on your usual breathing for 2-3 minutes at rest while sitting with a straight spine. What do you feel? If the sensations are vague, take a deep slow in-breath and slowly exhale. Do you feel how the airflow goes through your nostrils? Do you have any sensations at the back of your throat? Are there any feelings about movement of air inside the chest and bronchi? What do you sense near your stomach?

Usually, children have a good perception about their own breathing. Older people notice fewer sensations. Having these sensations makes the process of learning easier. However, even if the student feels nothing at all (rare, but possible), it is still possible to learn the method. How? First, the student can restore the sensations by doing special exercises and focusing his attention on his own breathing. Second, if these exercises do not work, as in very rare cases, the teacher can use, for the right students, special breathing exercises that do not need the feeling of one's breath.

To restore the sensations of your own breath, the following exercises can be used.

1. Put your hands around your waist line, as if embracing yourself, and listen to your usual breathing for about 20-30 seconds. You will be able to detect the movements of the diaphragm.

2. Put your hands slightly (about 10 cm or 4 inches higher) around your waist and listen to your usual breathing for about 20-30 seconds. You will be able to detect the movements of the rib cage.

In most cases, repeating these exercises a few times will solve the problem. If the sensations are still not present, the student should practice the exercise with the books and the exercise with the belt described below.

Stage 2: Relaxation of the body's muscles

The student is asked to tense some parts of his body muscles and then relax them. This is usually not a problem for a particular arm or leg, but is more difficult when more muscles are involved. To learn tension and relaxation of the whole body gradually, the student can start with some muscles and then add other groups.

For our future goals, the student should be able:

- to tense the whole body and then relax it

- to tense the upper part of the body (from the rib cage up) and then relax it.

Section 4.14 of this chapter provides additional relaxation techniques related to the visualization of relaxation.

Stage 3: Tensing and relaxing breathing muscles

As a next logical step, the student tries to tense and relax the breathing muscles, which we divide, for our purposes, into 2 groups:

- the diaphragm (other names are "tummy", "belly", and "stomach")

- all remaining breathing muscles (other names are "chest muscles", "rib cage muscles", and "thoracic muscles").

Here all these muscles are tensed and relaxed together. In order to achieve success, do the following simple exercise. Close the mouth and stop breathing through the nose (using our throat lock mechanism). Try to take a strong and big inhale, while there is no way for the air to move into the lungs. This helps to achieve a strong sensation of tension in the breathing muscles. Keep the tension for 1-2 seconds and then relax the muscles and take light inhalation.

Stage 4: Considered separately as a Buteyko breathing exercise

4.6 Relaxing the diaphragm (Buteyko relaxed breathing exercise)

This Section of the book provides the safest diaphragmatic breathing exercise (relaxed diaphragmatic breathing).

Relaxed diaphragmatic breathing is the main exercise for people with hypertension and other forms of heart disease to lower their heart rate (pulse) and gradually reduce their blood pressure. Bear in mind that many hypertensives, when they have less than 20 s for the body oxygen test, are not able to get benefits from regular Buteyko breathing exercises that involve breath holds and reduced breathing.

However, even if you do not have problems with hypertension and panic attacks, you can still get benefits from reading and practicing this exercise.

Can you breathe for 1-2 minutes using the tummy or stomach only? If you are uncertain or your sensations are absent or vague, it is necessary to review Chapter 1 (Diaphragmatic breathing).

If you are able to breathe using mainly the diaphragm (while sitting with a straight spine and being at rest), the next step is to learn how to relax the diaphragm during exhalations. (Note: if you can achieve abdominal, but not diaphragmatic breathing, you are still doing great and are ready for the next step.)

Advanced Buteyko Breathing Exercises

Each exhale should be accompanied by the relaxation of all bodily muscles. The changes in the breathing pattern for a person with the low initial CP, who practices relaxation of the diaphragm only (no deliberate air hunger), are shown below.

Buteyko relaxed breathing exercise

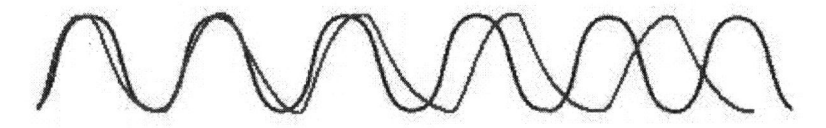

www.NormalBreathing.com

Your breathing before this exercise is shown using the black line (with forceful exhalations). During this exercise (the blue line), you should try to unblock the diaphragm or at least have abdominal breathing. You have the following goal: take your usual inhalation using your diaphragm only and then relax your diaphragm for exhalation. This will make your exhalations smooth (the blue line for your new breathing pattern). Note that the depth of your inhalations remains the same, but the frequency of your breathing becomes smaller. Hence, reduced breathing for low CP students is achieved using relaxation only. If you do this exercise correctly, you should notice that your pulse or heart rate is lower after a session that lasts more than 10 minutes. (We are going to discuss durations of breathing exercises later.)

For most people, this is a transitory (temporary) exercise. (Heart and hypertension patients should stick with this exercise until they get over 20 s CP and reduce or lower their high blood pressure to normal levels without medication.)

If you do not have hypertension or panic attacks, you can practice this exercise for 2-3 minutes so that you get a clear sensation of your relaxed diaphragmatic exhalation. (You can or even should wear the belt during this exercise, if you are not sure about your ability to breathe using your diaphragm only. The belt will prevent you from any chest breathing. Its use is described above in Chapter 1.)

People with very low CPs (less than 10 seconds) may find that they have very frequent breathing during this exercise and are unable to get relaxation. In such cases, you should make the inhalations short and sharp (as if you are sniffing air and have very short but active inhalations). Then you will have more time to relax all body muscles and have longer inhalations.

4.7 Buteyko reduced breathing exercise with light air hunger

Detailed instructions for RB (reduced breathing) exercise, Dr. Buteyko instruction (formula for the RB in a nutshell), and typical sensations and signs indicating that the students indeed breathe less air.

After previous easy exercises, you should be able to consciously create and maintain light air hunger while breathing little less air using the diaphragm (or abdominal muscles) and relax all breathing and body muscles for exhalations. Let us review the process of the RB (reduced breathing) in more detail.

If your CP is below 20 s, follow these instructions:

Instead of taking a big and deep inhalation, take a slightly smaller inhalation (only about 5-10% less than your usual inhalation) using the diaphragm and then immediately relax all muscles, especially all breathing muscles. Then immediately, repeat the same: take a (smaller) inhalation and again completely relax.

Buteyko Reduced Breathing for less than 20 s CP

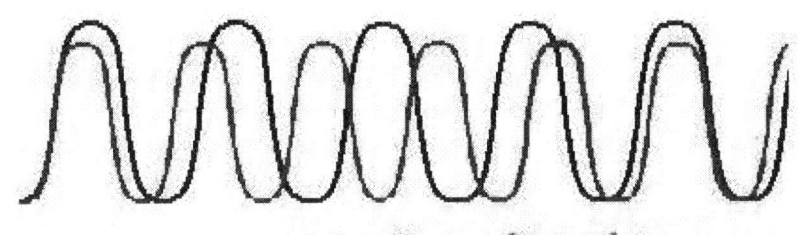

www.NormalBreathing.com

The blue line in this picture shows the pattern of RB for people with low CPs (less than 20 s). The black line is your breathing pattern just before the exercise.

If you practice this exercise, in 1-2 minutes you will experience light air hunger (or light desire to breathe more). Your initial goal is to preserve this light comfortable level of air hunger for about 5 minutes.

It is normal that breathing is frequent during your reduced or shallow breathing. The crucial thing is that you breathe less, your inhalations are less deep, and you are relaxed.

If your CP is 20 s or more, follow these instructions:

If one's CP is above 20 s, then the pattern of RB (reduced breathing) is usually different. Why? Because usual breathing, while resting or sleeping, is also different. For example, if the actual CP is about 30 s, the student is likely to have short automatic pauses (about 1 s) or total relaxation (no breathing) after exhalations. These automatic pauses are individual and also depend on the actual personal CP. The higher the CP, the longer the automatic pause. Presence of longer automatic pauses is a sign of better health.

While practicing the RB, the students with higher CPs (over 20 s) not only slightly reduce their inhalations but, in addition, they can have short periods of total relaxation with no breathing.

Buteyko Reduced Breathing for about 25 s CP

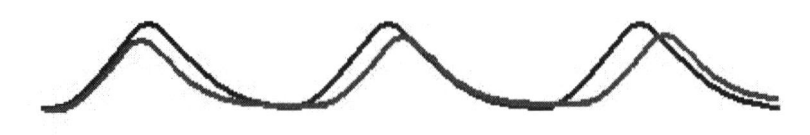

www.NormalBreathing.com

This figure shows reduced breathing (represented by the blue line) when the CP is about 25 s. First, inhalations are smaller than the original ones (the black line shows breathing before the exercise); second, the durations of exhalations and pauses of total relaxation are longer. Hence, you breathe slightly less air and also slightly slower.

The 20 s CP threshold also separates relatively healthy people with over 20 s CP who have an automatic pause (even during automatic breathing) and sick people with less than 20 s CP who do not have this automatic pause.

More details about the reduced breathing

The RB should cause light shortage of air (air hunger) in about 1-2 minutes. It requires some experimentation from the student to find out the depth of inhalations and durations of automatic pauses (no breathing).

For example, with about 20 s CP, one's RB probably does not require any pauses. Each subsequent inhalation immediately follows the previous exhalation, as described in the previous section.

Advanced Buteyko Breathing Exercises

If your CP is about 30 s, you can take a smaller inhale, relax for the exhalation and can enjoy total relaxation for about 2-3 seconds (no breathing movements). Then this cycle is repeated again and again, until the student gets slight air hunger. Once the right breathing pattern is found (so that you can maintain light air hunger for 5-10 minutes or more), do mental counting (e.g., "one, two, three") for automatic pauses after each exhalation. The structure of your breathing can be presented using the following description:
Shorter inhale – Relax all muscles for the exhalation – Slow mental counting, "One, two, three" (total rest) –
Shorter inhale – Relax all muscles for the exhalation – Slow mental counting, "One, two, three" (total rest) –
Shorter inhale – Relax all muscles for the exhalation – Slow mental counting, "One, two, three" (total rest) –
Shorter inhale – Relax all muscles for the exhalation – Slow mental counting, "One, two, three" (total rest) –

When the CP gets larger, the durations of automatic pauses at rest and during this exercise are also increased. For example, with 40 s CP, the student can usually have about a 5-6 s pause after each exhalation during the whole RB period. With 60 s CP, the pause gets up to about 10 s for total relaxation, and so forth. Mental counting is useful, but not necessary.

Your next step (for people with any CP): practice the RB for about 5 minutes

When you practice the RB for 1-2 minutes, you should get a light feeling of air hunger (you want to breathe more but resist the desire and teach your own body to have lighter breathing). The key of the exercise is to maintain this shallow (or reduced), diaphragmatic breathing pattern for about 5 minutes with relaxation of all muscles and a light hunger for air.

Another practical suggestion, which was emphasized by Dr. Buteyko, is that under no circumstances is it allowed to have large deep inhalations or quick exhalations during the RB. Breathing, especially exhalations, should be under full control and totally relaxed. You do nothing for exhalation, just relax all body muscles.

Every time you get a desire to take a deep breath by chest expansion, calmly and consistently relax all muscles, especially chest-shoulders-neck-jaw muscles, and continue to breathe less using the diaphragm.

The level of air hunger during the RB session should be light and comfortable, no more than at the end of the CP, (it is felt, but comfortable enough and easy to tolerate). During the first breathing sessions this sensation of air hunger is unusual and, for some people, unpleasant. Meanwhile, after realizing the relaxing and inspiring effects of the first sessions, these unpleasant effects disappear.

Possible mistake: you breathe too little

Occasionally, a student is so motivated to breathe less that they start to breathe too little, e.g., 2 times less than before the RB. This may be possible for about 2-3 minutes only. But the body needs to adjust to any level of breathing gradually. Hence, later the degree of biochemical stress (due to CO_2 increase) for the body can be so high, that it will be impossible to suppress very deep and heavy gasps for air. Therefore, for initial stages of learning, keep the level of air hunger light and comfortable.

How Dr. Buteyko described the essence of the RB

The manual written by Dr. Buteyko (Buteyko, 1991), in order to remember the essence of the Buteyko method (shallow or reduced breathing), suggests to use the rule of "The left hand". *"This rule contains 5 points (5 fingers, starting from the thumb):*
1. decrease
2. the depth
3. of breathing
4. by relaxation of the diaphragm
5. till slight shortage of air" (Buteyko, 1991).

Advanced Buteyko Breathing Exercises

The last point, according to Dr. Buteyko, is the most difficult to learn.

In other words, take smaller diaphragmatic inhalations with relaxed exhalations and a sensation of light air hunger.

Note that the frequency of breathing is not important in the Buteyko method. Breathing less with the relaxed diaphragm is the key. Buteyko breathing consists of a shallow, low-tidal-volume voluntary breathing pattern.

Review of the main factors

In short, the main factors of RB are:
- smaller inhalations using the diaphragm only;
- passive and relaxed exhalations (no efforts are applied, and all body muscles are relaxed in order to produce exhalations);
- light air hunger;
- thorough relaxation of all body muscles;
- correct body posture;
- comfortably cool environment;
- good air quality;
- empty stomach (water is OK);
- nasal breathing only and no speaking.

Each of these conditions is crucial for success.

Signs and symptoms of success: what would you feel during and after the correct RB?

If you breathe less, during the RB period, you will notice the following signs:
- The arms and feet will get warm in about 2-3 minutes after starting the RB (this is the central and most important sign present in over 90% students who practice it correctly).
- The nasal passages will be clearer (especially when the nose was partly blocked before).
- The nose will often become a little more moist and cold in about

the same 2-3 minutes. (However, this effect will not take place if the air quality is unsuitable for you or if you have chronic problems with sinuses and nasal breathing.)
- The diaphragm will become slightly tense and unsettled. Indeed, if you breathe less, your breathing center tries to intensify respiration, while you are doing the opposite job: teaching the breathing center how to breathe less.

There are many other individual and occasional signs and symptoms indicating that the student breathes less:
- tears in eyes;
- increased salivation;
- restoration of the muscular tone of the transverse colon and stomach leading to the natural desire to sit straight;
- the desire to flex and stretch arms (especially after the session);
- feeling of increased energy (or feeling of being charged);
- feeling of being focused (instead of confused and indecisive);
- reduced hunger for food and addictive substances, etc.

You may have some of these additional symptoms or none of them. However, increased feeling of energy and improved concentration are very common signs.

4.8 Using reduced breathing for symptoms, sleep, and bowel movements

Once you have learned reduced breathing, you need to apply it for various real-life situations in order to see its healing power.

For example, many people strain themselves in order to have **bowel movements**. This is not a healthy practice. In order to have easy and natural bowel movements, you need to apply reduced breathing. And this can be done for all bowel movements (unless you have diarrhea or bowel movements are easy for you). Most people with chronic constipation are able get rid of this symptom in less than 1 minute if they apply breath holding with reduced breathing.

Advanced Buteyko Breathing Exercises

The next effective application of reduced breathing is for **falling asleep fast**. It is very common for modern people to spend up to 10-15 minutes in bed when they try to fall asleep. With reduced breathing, it is much easier. The time that is required to fall asleep is often reduced up to 3-7 times. The same is true if you wake up at night or suffer from insomnia.

Many people suffer from **sleepiness after meals**. When you get sleepy while digesting food, the most likely cause is a lack of good chewing and eating too much (overeating). In this case, you cannot and should not practice reduced breathing, but you need to change your eating habits. When you get sleepy after the meal is digested, then breath holding and reduced breathing will help you to become energetic and alert in 1-2 minutes.

There are many other symptoms that can be easily solved with reduced breathing. They include situation when you need to solve the following challenges:
- how to stop coughing
- how to get rid of a stuffy nose
- how to stop a runny nose
- how to warm hands and feet
- how to stop panic attacks and anxiety
- how to stop asthma attacks
- how to stop heart attacks
- and many others.

Nearly all people (unless someone has contraindications and restrictions outlined above) can do a breath hold before doing reduced breathing. This helps to achieve the desirable effects faster.

4.9 Your daily log for breathing exercises and how to fill it

Your main breathing retraining daily log (or your personal breath-work diary) for Buteyko breathing exercises (and for practicing with breathing devices too) can be freely found online in the Downloads Section of NormalBreathing.com. You can get different type formats: a Rich Text Format file and an Excel spreadsheet (if you want to fill your daily log digitally on your PC), or a PDF file (for printing).

Practice of successful students shows that it is very important to keep records of your progress.

For example, in order to solve the problem of morning hyperventilation (and this is the problem for over 80% of all breathing students), the daily log and knowledge about the extent of this problem in your particular case is vital. Whatever you want to check (your real requirements in essential fatty acids, Ca, and Mg; your sensitivity to carpets, the effects of physical exercise on your CP growth), the daily log, if correctly filled, will reflect the effects of these factors on your main health parameters: the CP and pulse. Even if you want to test various versions of Buteyko breathing exercises, you will find the daily log beneficial.

Here are several lines from one daily log.

Advanced Buteyko Breathing Exercises

Date	Morn CP	Time (hour)	Initial pulse	Initial CP	Breath cycle or RB session time	Final pulse	Final CP	Physic. activity	Symptoms, medication and auxiliary activities
7.05	-	1 pm	76	16	12 s, 17 s - 12 m	72	22	40 min	8 am - ventolin 2 puffs
		5 pm	76	17	11 s, 16 s - 12 m	74	20		tight chest
		11 pm	74	16	13 s, 15 s - 12 m	70	24		
8.05	12	9 am	78	18	14 s, 18 s - 12 m	76	22	45 min	Taped mouth
		4 pm	72	17	12 s, 18 s - 12 m	70	21		overnight - no ventolin
		10 pm	74	18	14 s, 17 s - 12 m	70	27		

Each line represent one breathing session (in this case, all of them are 12 min long). The very first column is the **Date**. So, write the date.

The next column is the **Morning CP** or the result of the CP test immediately after waking up. (You need to learn and know how to measure the morning CP and why it is important.)

Then we have the approximate time of the day when you do the breathing session (the **"Time (hour)"** column).

The next column is your **Initial pulse**. You can use any device to define your current heart rate or do it yourself. The pulse is usually measured at the wrist area using 2 or 3 fingers of the other hand. Or you may measure your pulse on your neck (find the depression near the thyroidal gland that allows you to feel the carotid artery leading to the brain) or chest. There is no need to measure the heart rate during one minute, but 10, 15 and 20 s intervals are not long enough since changes in pulse (before and after breathing sessions) are small. We do pulse counting during a 30 s interval. Then multiply the number of heart beats by 2 and you get your pulse in one minute. This number is to be filled in the daily log.

The next parameter to record is the **Initial CP**.

As you see from this log, the reduced breathing is the next step and it starts immediately after the initial CP. This is the main part of the session. You can see that the daily log includes 2 intermediate breath holds (for the first row, they are 12 and 17 s long), while the duration of the reduced breathing was 12 min (**Session time**).

After the reduced breathing, you measure your **Final pulse** and, after 2-3 min of rest, you measure your **Final CP**. (The fact that you need to rest is also mentioned in the note at the bottom of the daily log, but this part is not shown above.) Why do we need this short break? We cannot measure the final CP immediately after the RB since you may still have air hunger. But in 2-3 min this air hunger will be lost and we can find parameters related to your new breathing pattern

Advanced Buteyko Breathing Exercises

and new level of body oxygenation. This is the end of the breathing session.

The daily log also includes the amount of your **Physical activity** (in minutes) and the column about your **Symptoms, medication and auxiliary activities**. In short, anything that can influence your health and breathing should be shown in this last column.

4.10 Structure and effects of one breathing session

The most common Buteyko breathing session has the following structure:
Initial Pulse Test - Initial CP Test - RB (for 3-5 minutes) - Intermediate breath hold - RB (for 3-5 minutes) -
..
- Intermediate breath hold - RB (for 3-5 minutes) -
- Intermediate breath hold - RB (for 3-5 minutes) - Pulse Test - 2-3 min rest - Final CP Test

The total duration of one such session can range from 12 up to 30-35 minutes (if you have light air hunger).

The periods of reduced breathing are 3-5 minutes long.

These periods of reduced breathing are followed by intermediate breath holds. Their purpose is to remind you about air hunger. Note that it is normal that intermediate breath holds are shorter than the initial CP (because they are done when you already have air hunger). The duration of the RB periods depend on the duration of intermediate breath holds and the CP:
When the CP is short (e.g., less than 20 s), choose 3-4 min for each cycle.
When the CP is between 20 and 40 s, choose 4 min for each cycle.
When the CP is more than 40 s, choose 5 min for each cycle.

This graph illustrates the structure of one breathing session with light air hunger and 4 min of reduced breathing.

Breathing exercise with slight air hunger

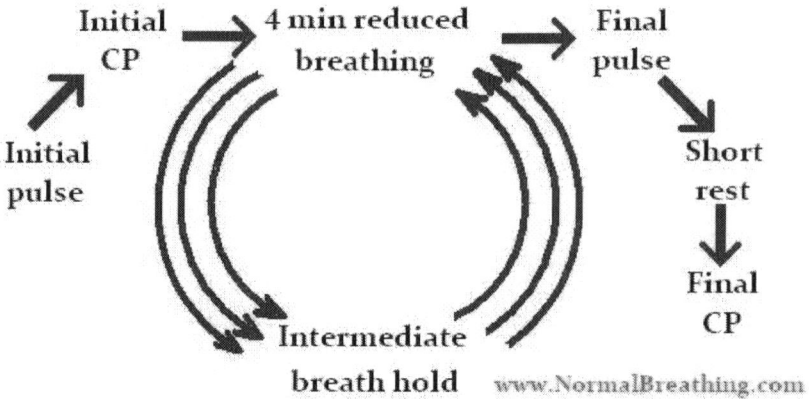

Initial CP → 4 min reduced breathing → Final pulse

Initial pulse

Intermediate breath hold

Short rest

Final CP

www.NormalBreathing.com

In this particular example, the duration of one cycle (that includes breath holding and reduced breathing) is 4 minutes. In other words, you have intermediate breath holds each 4 minutes. This means that, for this breathing session, you do intermediate breath holds 3 times: at 4, 8 and 12 minutes.

If your CP and intermediate breath holds are about 20 seconds, then the durations of reduced breathing are about 3 minutes 40 seconds. But for the sake of simplicity, we may say that you do reduced breathing for 4 minutes. In reality, the duration of each cycle on this chart is 4 minutes, while the duration of the breathing exercise (how long you control your breath) is 16 minutes. The whole session takes little more time since you need to measure and record initial and final parameters. In this case, you will need 19-20 minutes in total to complete this breathing session.

When should you practice breathing exercises?

A. When you have unpleasant symptoms due to hyperventilation (wheezing, chest tightness, anxiety, cold hands and feet, constipation, insomnia, headaches, etc.). In such cases, you need only an Emergency Procedure that is usually about 3-5 min long, but, in severe cases, can be over 10 minutes.

Advanced Buteyko Breathing Exercises

B. As a part of your daily program (and this is what the daily log is for) to increase the CP. In such cases, you do the whole session.

What are the main criteria of success for one breathing session?

1. The most important criterion is your easier or lighter breathing after the session. **Your final CP should be at least by 5 s greater than the initial CP and you should view your CP increase as your main goal for any session.** (Remember, that the final CP is measured 2-3 minutes after finishing the RB. But you can also measure it 10 or 30 minutes after the session and the CP should still be higher than your initial CP).

2. The pulse (or heart rate) usually drops by about 2-3 beats per minute or more after the session. Occasionally it can get higher, especially if you drank coffee or ate chocolate before the session. Hence, you need to monitor the heart rate drop and experience this effect for most of your sessions.

3. The arms and feet will get warm in about 2-3 minutes after starting the RB.

Most of my students are able to get the RB right from the first attempt and they consistently experience all 3 major signs of success described above: warmer hands and feet soon after starting the RB, a higher final CP and lower final pulse (after the session). A small number of people may consistently have a higher CP and higher pulse after correct breathing sessions. Also keep in mind that, as mentioned above, caffeine and chocolate can increase your *final* pulse.

Breathing exercises are beneficial when you experience all 3 signs in 90% of all your breathing sessions. For example, assume that you completed 10 breathing sessions. Then you can analyze your daily log and find out the emerging pattern. If you got all 3 signs in 9 sessions out of 10, this is an excellent result. If you got 7-8 sessions right, it is still not bad, but you should figure out what was wrong with the remaining 2-3 breathing sessions. If you succeed only in 6 or fewer sessions, you should stop these breathing exercises and find some fundamental reason of your failure. Do not waste your time on something that does not consistently improve your body oxygenation and the CP.

During last year, I found that it is much easier for my students with low initial CPs (less than 20 s) to learn how to practice with the Frolov or Amazing DIY Breathing device first, increase the daily CP up to about 20-25 s, and then learn the Buteyko exercises. In my view, it is the optimum approach to breathing retraining: start with the DIY device, get up to about 20-25 s at least, and then learn RB and other, more advanced Buteyko exercises.

If there are no improvements

Practice shows that these three major signs (higher CP, lower pulse, and warmer hands and feet) are all present or absent together. Hence, when you already have done several breathing sessions, it will be clear if you get them or not. If they are not present, you need to stop and think about the causes. Even if only half of your breathing sessions are successful (all 3 signs are there), it is necessary to search for the causes.

Most likely, something is wrong with one or more of the initial parameters of the exercises. Here is a check-list of questions:

• Do you have a **comfortably cool environment**? Remember you should not feel warm during exercises. If your CP is less than 20 s, keep yourself at a normal temperature or even slightly warm. If your CP is more than 20 s and you do not have a cold/viral infection, keep yourself on a slightly cool side. If you have on too many clothes or practice in a too warm surrounding temperature, no progress should be expected. Also, direct sunlight, causing heating of one side of your body and mild cellular damage due to penetrating radiation, is another factor to avoid.

• Is the **air quality** good enough for you? If you are sensitive or allergic to any chemical or substance in the air, you will not be able

Advanced Buteyko Breathing Exercises

to slow down your breathing. Air born particles can increase the area and degree of inflammation depleting your cortisol reserves and causing other negative effects. Try to do some breathing exercises in ideal conditions: outdoors, in a park, the backyard of your house, or in the kitchen with the windows open, etc. in order to see the effects.

• Do you always do exercises with **no solid food in the stomach**? Generally, as it was emphasized by Dr. Buteyko, only water does not intensify respiration.

• Are you sufficiently hydrated? Remember to **drink water** at first signs of thirst.

• Do you maintain a **correct body posture** during the session? The higher your CP, the stronger the effect of a correct posture on your breathing and CP. When your CP is about 25 s, a poor posture will definitely prevent you from further CP increase. When the CP gets beyond 20 s, a correct posture is vital for further progress.

• Do you take **smaller inhalations during the RB**? If you breathe more and do not have light comfortable air hunger with little more CO2 in the lungs, your parameters (the CP and pulse) will not improve.

• Do you **use only your diaphragm for inhalations**? If you are unsure, use a belt, as described above, so as to suppress any chest movements.

• How do you **exhale** air during the RB? Do you just **relax all your body**, including all breathing muscles? Exhalations require relaxation only, but, when the CP is low, this element of the RB also requires attention. If you push air out forcefully, you can easily hyperventilate and become tenser.

• Do you experience **light comfortable air hunger** that is easy to tolerate and maintain for 12 or more minutes?

- Do you constantly remind yourself to **relax all body muscles**? If you focus too much on diaphragmatic inhalations and light air hunger, muscles, especially in the upper part of the body, can get tense making lighter breathing difficult or impossible. Being totally relaxed and having light air hunger are the most challenging parts of the Buteyko breathing exercises.

- Various **fears (conscious, subconscious, and unconscious)** lead to spasm of blood vessels and increased muscular tension. It can be impossible to slow down breathing when fears are present. Are you able to leave or separate all your irrelevant worries from your breathing retraining activities? In some cases, the reduction of anxiety (fears are indeed groundless) and different attitudes are more effective than relaxation exercises. Easier breathing and higher CPs will help you to have a much more realistic picture of the real world. Fears may also exist in relation to the pauses, feeling of air hunger, or some other attributes of the method, the exercises, surrounding people or the whole environment. Do you have sufficient confidence, trust and faith that breathing retraining can reduce or eliminate your health symptoms? If you spent too little time on educational topics on breathing, these spiritual and psychological parameters of your motivation can suffer.

- If you are **deficient in cortisol** your parameters after the session will be almost unchanged. You may not be able to increase your CP, if you suffer from any inflammatory condition and related problems (such as asthma, bronchitis, arthritis, IBD, various digestive problems, cystic fibrosis, cancer, etc.), adrenal exhaustion, severe and chronic stress and that your current CP is less than 20 s. Cortisol, in cases of deficiency, according to Dr. Buteyko and his colleagues, is vital for breathing normalization. No progress is possible unless you provide what the body needs to fight inflammation, infection, and stress. There is a separate module devoted to cortisol deficiency (if not online, then in projects).

- If you are **severely obese**, you will likely be stuck with a low CP (less than 20 s) for a longer time in comparison with people who have nearly normal body weight. It will be difficult, during the breathing session, to increase your CP even by 1-2 seconds, but breathing exercises will reduce your hunger and provide you with more energy. It is crucial, in such conditions, to follow the natural desire to eat less and only low-calorie foods. Very long walks and other light forms of physical exercise with 100% nasal breathing (in and out) will greatly help you to progress faster.

• If you are **genetically predisposed to cardiovascular problems, migraines, and panic** attacks, you will experience unpleasant symptoms, like dizziness, mild headache, fog in the head, strange sensations of thirst, etc. Then you should be able or even can notice that you feel better while doing the RB without breath holds. You should practice different breathing exercises with a very gradual CO2 increase.

4.11 Some questions and answers about breathing exercises and the CP test

Q: My CP increases and pulse goes down after the breathing session, but arms and feet remain cold. Is something wrong?
A: This usually happens in cases of chronic problems with circulation, Raynaud's disease, etc., when the CP is less than 20 s. It is great that your CP is growing. Once you get more than 20 s CP, you will notice changes in your sensation of warmth in arms and feet.

Q: I can increase my CP by more than 5 s and my arms and feet do become warm. However, my heart rate often increases, especially after the morning breathing sessions, since I drink several cups of coffee. Should I stop drinking coffee?
A: Coffee helps many low-CP people to be more alert and function better. Hence, drink coffee, if it improves your life and performance. When your morning CP will be over 30 s, your desire to drink coffee will be naturally reduced or can completely disappear because your energy level, focus, and concentration will greatly improve. Then drinking coffee will start to produce heart palpitations and other negative effects. The same relates to chocolate, cocoa, strong tea and other caffeine-containing products.

Q: Should I try to control my respiratory rate during a breathing session?
A: Dr. Buteyko, during one of his lectures for the staff members of the Moscow State University, said, "But the breathing frequency is strictly individual: it depends on gender, age, weight, etc., and, as a rule, it is not limited. We prohibit the sick to think about it, otherwise it would confuse them." He, after continuous observation of patients, also found that, with time, the breathing center automatically adjusts the breathing rate to the existing arterial CO_2 level. With a higher CP, people generally breathe less frequently naturally. You can check this phenomenon. Ask your relative to measure your breathing frequency at night or when you are at rest. However, the way you practice breathing exercises is a factor that can influence your respiratory rate months or years later.

Q: Why is it necessary to wait for 2-3 minutes to measure the final CP after the RB?
A: The goal of the session is to reduce your breathing and breathe less during the next hours. Hence, we should measure the after-effect of the session. If the student measures the final CP immediately after the RB, he or she still has air hunger and the value would be smaller than after 2-3 minutes of rest. After sufficient rest with no breathing control, the CP reflects your improvements in oxygenation. Usually the CP is measured after 2-3 minutes of rest, but one can measure the final CP even later: 5, 10 or even 30 minutes after the session.

Q: Can I do my first daily breathing session soon or immediately after waking up?
A: This depends on your evening and morning CPs. For example, if you wake up and your CP is almost the same as the evening CP, you will not be able to further reduce breathing (it is better to do some physical exercise in this case). However, if your morning CP is much less than the evening CP (e.g., you have 20 s CP in the evening, but only 10 s CP in the morning), then breathing exercises will help you to restore your oxygenation. Then having an early breathing session is a right step.

Advanced Buteyko Breathing Exercises

Q: I have little time for the breathing exercises. Can I start them without preliminary rest for 3-5 minutes? Does it affect my initial CP?
A: When a person is in a rush, the first CP is measured soon after physical activity. That can reduce the initial CP and may cause more anxiety and tension (since you have less time to relax your mind), but you may still get the main benefits of breathing exercises.

Q: I try really hard and had over 10 breathing sessions, but my CP is 11-12 seconds and stays like a rock. What is wrong?
A: This is rare, and there are many explanations. You can be deficient in some essential nutrients, or cortisol-deficient, or suffer from severe obesity, or have several serious health problems, etc.. You require more professional help. You can send me your daily log and meet me for an online lesson.

Q: Sometimes I feel that my neck or jaws are too tense. Is small muscular tension a serious problem?
A: There is an intimate link between any muscular tension and breathing. On the one hand, hyperventilation causes tense muscles as a normal and useful evolutionary response to a "fight or flight" situation. On the other hand, chronic hyperventilators are tense all the time. That can be observed in their posture, walking and other activities. Being relaxed is a difficult problem for them and is something that they need to learn. Normal breathing, on the other hand, is characterized by normal CO_2 concentrations. Since CO_2 is a powerful relaxant of body muscles, reduced breathing leads to natural relaxation. That is also the reason why people feel calm and relaxed after the Buteyko breathing exercises.

From a practical viewpoint, it is indeed very important to eliminate all unnecessary muscular tension. For that reason, various relaxation exercises, meditation, massage, yoga postures, Alexander technique, all are useful in breathing normalization.

Q: While practicing the Buteyko breathing exercises, should I keep my jaws (and teeth) clenched together or they can be slightly open?
A: Keeping the jaw muscles totally relaxed, while making sure that

the mouth is closed, these are important factors for success. Therefore, relax your jaw muscles and all surrounding muscles as much as possible.

Q: I consistently get some muscular tension and unpleasant sensations in the jaw area after breathing exercises. Why is this so?
A: It is likely that easier breathing and higher CP activate some healing processes in your jaw and try to restore some tissues or fight pathogens there. You may have plaque on your teeth, too much food particles between teeth, mercury amalgams, cavities in teeth, root canals, gingivitis, or some other abnormalities. Remove the plaque, regularly floss and brush your teeth, try strong mouth wash (to check its effects on this symptom), and do other activities related to dental hygiene and the elimination of possible focal infections.

Q: Can the Buteyko method help me with my poor body posture and prolapse of the colon?
A: Since the Buteyko breathing normalizes blood flow, the oxygenation and tone of the large intestine, some people normally feel that breathing sessions naturally help them to correct the curvature of their spine. They often experience a desire to sit, stand and walk with the correct body posture after breathing sessions. Therefore, Buteyko breathing is a powerful method to naturally correct the prolapse of the colon. Correction of a possible Mg deficiency can also greatly improve one's posture and prolapse of the colon.

Q: I am very confused about one thing. Some people recommend doing many breathing sessions during the day, others only two. Some recommend as many as I can; some say that too many is bad. I read in the book by James Hooper that the more I do the RB the faster my progress, but some people tell me that I cannot do more than 4 sessions a day? Why they all say different opinions? Shouldn't the Buteyko method be always the same?
A: When we learn the method, we are different in respect to:
1) Hereditary parameters (the weak systems and organs of the body)
2) Actual or initial health states
3) Abilities, possibilities and motivation to learn the method.

Advanced Buteyko Breathing Exercises

Depending on these parameters the optimum plan can be chosen.

However, there are common ideas. You can have RB - with light air hunger- all the day (no pauses or only one long breath hold per hour.) You can do short sessions, 10-15 min of RB (with 2 CPs) every hour (e.g., when the clock strikes the hour - start the session), but not more often. You can do long sessions (about 25-30 min with 6-7 CPs per session) every 2 hours, but not more often. However, even here there are restrictions. Pregnant women, during certain stages and with low initial CPs, should not follow these suggestions due to their specific restrictions.

If you have hypertensions, panic attacks, or migraines, it is better not to do CPs, but only RB (as explained above). In very rare cases, the relaxation of the diaphragm for exhalations is the optimum activity during initial stages of health restoration.

The classic Buteyko method (practiced by Russian doctors in the 1970-80's) required more than 2-3 hours of breathing exercises per day.

Q: There are many activities and measures that can ensure good health. Eat right, exercise right, sleep right, do relaxation, maintain correct posture, use supplements, etc. Can I just lead a healthy life style without paying any special attention to breathing?
A: If you are healthy person and satisfied with the functioning of your organism (amazing vitality, excellent and short sleep, perfect digestion, etc.), than your breathing should be physiologically normal: your CP should be over 60 s CP naturally. Such people naturally breathe only through the nose during intensive exercise; they enjoy physical activity; they sleep no more than 4.5 hours without sleep restrictions, do not sleep on the back; they like to eat healthy and raw foods and have other health-promoting life parameters. Then you do not need any special breathing exercises.

However, if you are chronically sick and you are trying to restore your health using all natural methods (diet, exercise, relaxation, supplements, etc.), except breathing, it would take you much longer time, maybe years, in order to get healthy. The Buteyko method was specially designed for sick people so that they could quickly restore their normal breathing and regain vitality as soon as possible.

As about ordinary people without serious health problems, measure your CP to see where you are now.

Q.: When should the last daily set of breathing exercises (before going to sleep) be done?
A.: People report that the effects of the last breathing session can be slightly different depending on, for example, the timing and type of this breathing session. Therefore, find your optimum parameters. Some people do this last set about 2 hours before going to sleep, while others just before retirement. In addition, it is suggested to do the Emergency Procedure or the RB in bed, especially, if the bed is not warm enough, or if a student has cold hands or feet, or if a student is too stressed and anxious.

Q: Can I practice Buteyko exercises in warm or hot conditions?
A: We can get benefits from breathing exercises, when the surrounding temperature is no more than 21 degrees Celsius (or 70 degrees Fahrenheit). When the surrounding temperature is more than 21 degrees Celsius (70 degrees Fahrenheit), it is nearly impossible to slow down one's breathing and increase one's CP without special steps. For slightly warmer conditions, one can use a strong fan while doing breathing exercises in a T-shirt and shorts. As another method, or in addition to using a fan, you can try wearing a wet T-shirt in order to cool the body. Wearing a wet T-shirt can be combined with cooling due to a fan.

Another option is to do physical exercise instead of breathing exercises. Warm conditions will increase your perspiration. As a result, you get something that is similar to hot yoga. This solution will produce results that are compatible to a breathing session in colder conditions. For many people, physical exercise in hot conditions, due to sweating, can be even a more effective way to increase their CP.

4.12 Structure of the program of Buteyko breathing exercises

How much to exercise?

When Buteyko wrote his first manuals with the description of the method for medical doctors, he suggested **3-4 hours of breathing exercises every day**. This was the amount of training that he and his colleagues (over 150 Soviet medical doctors and other health professionals) recommended to their patients. Many of these patients were hospitalized and, therefore, had a lot of time and, in most cases, a strong desire to practice.

Patients who followed this rigorous program of breathing retraining, experienced quick and dramatic health improvements. In a typical situation, a former patient with numerous hospitalizations and using various medications in 3-6 months could jog and exercise rigorously while breathing through the nose, climb 5-7 floors up with mouth closed and no signs of the disease that kept him crippled for years.

What about those people who have little time but still want to learn the method? In other words, what is the minimum amount of daily practice so that there are positive changes in the right direction (breathing less)? The student should spend about 1 hour per day for breathing exercises in order to experience gradual improvements in breathing. (That has been my requirement for many years, which I mention when I teach groups. Note that due to strict adherence to positive lifestyle changes, my students usually get 3-5 s of CP growth in 1 week. With the use of the Frolov breathing device or the Amazing DIY breathing device, they often get up to 6-8 s CP increase in a week, while practicing slightly less than 1 hour.) One session lasts about 15-20 minutes. Hence, 3-4 sessions can be done every day. Or you can have 2 sessions that are 30 min long.

As mentioned above, have no more than 1 short breathing session every hour, or 1 long breathing session every 2 hours.

Possible daily structures of Buteyko breathing exercises

If you have a lot of free time and/or very motivated to learn fast:
- Practice 1 short breathing session (12 min long) every hour or
- Practice 1 long breathing session (about 25-30 min long) every 2 hours
- Practice reduced breathing all day long when you have no solid food in the stomach with no more than 1 breath hold each hour.

The minimum amount of breathing exercises for slow learners is 1 hour. To achieve this goal, you can:
- Practice 5 short sessions (12 min long) per day
- Practice 4 short sessions (15 min long) per day
- Practice 3 sessions (20 min long) per day, and spread them throughout the day (e.g., not all sessions in the morning)
- Practice 2 long sessions (30 min long) per day and spread them throughout the day for better overall effects.

Remember that the total amount of breath control (when you practice breath holds and reduced breathing together) is the key factor that defines your overall progress.

Personal persistence and self-discipline are the main tools for progress. It was not accidental that the Buteyko method was called in the USSR "willful liquidation of deep breathing" emphasizing the will power. (Some Russian patients invented the other, grotesque name "the Siberian method of self-suffocation".)

Severely sick students, as practice shows, are the most diligent students. However, most people on the West used and use a mild approach with 3-4 sessions per day that is easy and stress-free.

As during any learning process, expectations and standards established by the teacher are other important factors for progress. This also relates to the ability of the student to practice with no fear more intensively (for more time and with stronger air hunger) without any negative effects.

Day-after-day progress in breathing retraining

Advanced Buteyko Breathing Exercises

One's breathing remains easier and the CP higher for some hours after the session. Later, the influence of other factors (stress, meals, lack of physical activity, poor posture, etc.) will make breathing heavier and reduce the CP. However, the student does another session and the process of breathing retraining continues. This process and the dynamic of the CP, pulse and symptoms can be analyzed later.

Day after day, the CP usually does not increase steadily. During some days the typical CPs and the morning CP can be lower than during the previous day. However, if the student does at least 3-4 short sessions every day (about 1 hour in total), the CP will improve by **at least 2-3 s in a week time**.

As we discussed above, some students practice the RB all the time while awake or have up to 2-3 hours of breathing exercises per day. Such students often progress up to 5-10 s CP increase per week or even faster. This linear progress usually takes place until the student reaches about 35 for the morning CP. Then their morning CPs remain below 40 s for weeks, months or even years. Forty s CP is a very important threshold. Very few people are able to break through the 40 s MCP. When this happens, usually their morning CP suddenly increases up to 45 or more seconds. In other words, these students make a jump accompanied by numerous changes related to duration and quality of sleep, desire to exercise, and much more. Breaking through the MCP 40 relates to Level 3.

Gradualism: an approach to learning air hunger

When the novice starts to practice, it is important to understand that breath holds and any air hunger, in the lives of many people, are associated in the brain with extra-ordinary situations (e.g., suffocation or drowning). Hence, the mind, instead of getting alarmed, needs to learn how to accept breath holds and air hunger positively. This task is solved faster and easier, if the level of air hunger for first breathing sessions is so light that the student can keep all muscles of the body totally relaxed.

There are even more severe restrictions, in respect to air hunger, that are required for some people with, for example, a loss of CO_2 sensitivity, sleep apnea and heart disease. Their safest exercises are relaxation, progressive relaxation of the body and relaxation of the diaphragm without any voluntary changes in breathing and with no air hunger. Later, when the CP is about 20 - 25 s, even previously severely sick people can do the CP and practice RB with air hunger and no unpleasant effects.

Later, after many sessions, the nervous system will learn that there is no danger in breath holds and air hunger. Then the student can practice longer breath holds (extended pauses and maximum pauses) and comfortably accept intensive sessions with moderate and strong air hunger, if he or she found them more effective.

Conditioning the body to breath holds

The idea of a gradual increase in air hunger relates to another fundamental process. For a breathing student, the reaction of the body to breath holds gradually changes. From being a stress, breath holds become triggers of positive physiological changes, if this student practices breathing exercises correctly. What does this mean?

As we discussed above, during initial stages of learning, breath holds are stressful and cause breathing intensification. However, imagine that this student repeats the following process many thousands times: breath holding is followed by relaxation and reduced (easier) breathing. What would be the effect after months or years of practice? Of course, the body adapts or gets conditioned to this sequence of effects. Breath holds become a stimuli for relaxation and easier breathing.

The effect becomes particularly surprising and powerful when high CP students, after many months of practice, do longer breath holds, even maximum pauses. Indeed, one may expect that if they do 90 second Maximum Pause, they should have heavy breathing after it. In reality, after this long pause, only their first inhalation is larger than their usual inhalation, but their subsequent breathing naturally becomes light even without conscious efforts.

In my view, it is a beneficial effect that provides a great advantage in breaking through the 40 s MCP.

4.13 "Two hundred breath holds"

Some students are very busy with their lives and have no or too little time for formal Buteyko exercises. In such cases, they can practice many breath holds throughout the day followed by easy breathing. While the changes in the respiratory center are very small after a single breathing session, up to 100-200 breath holds per day can produce a sufficient impact on the breathing center to cause permanent positive changes.

This breathing exercise is often called "200 breath holds". The structure of this exercise is very simple: first, the students does the CP test and then about 30-60 s of reduced breathing in order to increase alveolar CO_2 to higher levels and produce a small impact on the breathing center. When the number of breath holds is large, the net effect can be large too. Let us have a little math here.

If the total duration of one session is only 1 minute (imagine a person who does 200 breath holds, about 20 seconds long, followed by 40 seconds of reduced breathing), then doing 200 breath holds throughout the day means 200 minutes of breathing exercises in total. This is 3 hours and 20 minutes of breath work. Obviously, these sessions are going to produce a very strong impact on the CP growth, and the student can get up to 7-10 s CP increase during first weeks of learning (or usually until they hit the 40 s morning CP threshold).

To have 200 short 1-min breathing sessions per day requires good motivation. We can also calculate that, if sleep takes about 7-8 hours and meals also require nearly the same 7-8 hours per day for digestion, then there are only 8-10 hours left for breathing exercises. For someone who has to do 200 breath holds within 10 hours, 20 breath holds are to be done each hour. This is the same as one breath hold each 3 minutes.

In my view, this exercise can fit well a group of people who have busy dynamic jobs (all the time on the move or walking) and who are very motivated to increase body oxygenation. I am not 100% certain if this exercise can be suitable for someone with a sitting job. In my view, it is not the best or even good option to sit for hours (even while practicing breathing exercises) without physical exercise if this person is able to exercise. Probably these are the main reasons why this breathing exercise is rarely used by Buteyko breathing teachers.

However, if you are very motivated to practice reduced breathing and to increase your CP fast to larger numbers, then this exercise can become the foundation of your progress and success. Even with about 100 short breathing sessions (1 min long each), a student still gets about 1 hour and 40 minutes of breathing exercises per day, usually enough to have a fast dynamic overall week-after-week progress.

4.14 Use of imagery

Visualization (also called imagery) is the name of the technique used in professional sport, during meditation, for elimination of stress and anxiety, and many other purposes. Over 90% of modern elite athletes apply imagery to increase their sport performance and achieve faster recovery.

In order to achieve better results and stronger effects, visualization relaxation can be used as an effective way to relax the mind and body muscles. We can achieve this goal:
1) by imagining how our muscles become relaxed using certain analogies and comparisons applied to different muscle groups of the whole body
2) by picturing a relaxing scene, such as a beach, peaceful forest, or any other serene place.

Clinical measurements confirmed that imagery produces an additional effect on tone of muscles and brain waves facilitating better relaxation and a more peaceful state of mind. These simple and tested ideas can be applied to more effective practice of the Buteyko breathing exercises.

4.15 Simple visualization applied to muscle groups

This is one of easiest methods that can be used during reduced breathing with any level of air hunger. (So far, we considered reduced breathing with a light air hunger, but imagery is beneficial for more advanced breathing exercises as well.)

Imagery relaxation exercise (instructions and script)

While practicing reduced breathing, relax your body by releasing all areas of tension. You can record this script and later play it during breathing sessions.

... Take a smaller abdominal inhalation... Relax your diaphragm and all other breathing muscles in order to exhale... Allow your legs to become soft and relaxed... Feel how feet and calves become calm and peaceful.

... Take a next reduced inhalation and immediately relax your breathing muscles, together with legs and feet... You feel how your lower legs become peaceful and relaxed.

... You make small abdominal inhalations... After these inhalations, you just relax all body muscles completely to exhale air without efforts.

... With each relaxed and small exhalation, imagine and feel a wave of relaxation... This waves flows from the soles of your feet, up to your ankles, and then to your hips and pelvic area.

... Your legs become soft, peaceful and relaxed, as soft as silk... Or imagine that your legs become as soft as cloud.

... You keep the legs relaxed... You have light and easy reduced breathing.... Now you focus on your body trunk... Your spine is straight, as a broom.

... Imagine how your straight spine becomes relaxed: first, at the bottom of the spine... Each vertebra at the bottom of your spine is relaxed... Inhalations are small... Exhalations are relaxed... You apply no efforts to exhale.

... Then you relax your middle spine. All muscles around middle vertebras become rested and relaxed.

... Finally, all vertebras and surrounding muscles, along your spine, from the tail bone up to the tip of your spine become relaxed... Small abdominal inhalations are followed by total relaxation... Your exhalations are passive, effortless, and easy.

... Muscles of your back, shoulders, and chest are all relaxed... These body parts are loosely hanging on your spine... Your spine is like a support or solid foundation for other body parts and organs... It allows you to have small abdominal inhalations and relaxed exhalations.

... Muscles of your back, shoulders, and chest also become soft, quiet, peaceful and relaxed: as soft as silk... Breathing is easy and small... Exhalations are passive and comfortable.

... Feel how your arms and legs are becoming loose and relaxed... Tension in arms and legs disappears...

A pleasant sensation of warmness and relaxation is felt in your hands... This warm sensation flows up to your lower arms, elbows, then upper arms, and finally shoulders.

... Your arms become soft, peaceful and relaxed, as soft as silk... You have small abdominal inhalations... They are followed by total relaxation... Your exhalations are effortless and easy.

Advanced Buteyko Breathing Exercises

... Relax your shoulders, neck and back by completely relaxing your spine. The upper part of your body becomes relaxed.

... Muscles of your jaws and face become peaceful and relaxed. Your jaw, muscles around your cheek and eyes, and the forehead become relaxed... Light small abdominal inhalations are followed by total relaxation of the body muscles, breathing muscles included.

... Visualize how your body releases all the tension... It becomes calm and relaxed... Breathing is small and easy.

You can practice reduced breathing while using this script. I plan to make audio recordings for various breathing exercises in 2013. Some of these recordings should include all steps required for one breathing session (with recording of the initial pulse, initial CP, intermediate breath holds, and so forth). Other recording may provide only the relaxation scripts. You can check NormalBreathing.com for presence of these audio scripts.

You can also use the above script as a preparatory step for the next step: the imagery of scenes that can produce even better relaxation.

4.16 Imagery of scenes for better relaxation

The next step is to use the imagery of scenes during reduced breathing. The imagery or visualization of various scenes from nature helps to produce even better relaxation as documented in clinical studies that measured the effects of such methods on the tone of muscles, brain waves, and other bodily parameters.

However, in order to get maximum benefits from imagery, the person needs to achieve the following effect: visual images should be recreated in the mind together with effects related to other senses (smell, sounds, and so on). This means that, in addition to a visual picture, it is useful to experience accompanying sensations. For example, when you try to visualize yourself lying on a beach, you should also imagine a breeze from the ocean, warm rays of the sun, sounds of waves, and so forth.

As about the viewpoint for your visual picture, there are two approaches. Some people say that seeing yourself from outside or seeing yourself as you would see yourself in real life produce the same result. However, other people claim that seeing yourself in the same way as you see yourself in real life is more effective. This view is probably correct. Therefore, try to see your body the same way as you would see it in real life (not from outside).

Imagery works better if your visual pictures are present in your mind in colors (i.e., not black and white).

... Imagine you are lying on the beach... You can see and hear the waves crashing to the shore... You see the bright blue-green ocean spreading to the horizon with ships and yacht miles away from you... Your body muscles become light and relaxed... Tension and stiffness of muscles gradually disappear... Your breathing becomes small and very light.

... You see the blue sky with birds flying high in the sky... You close your eyes, and make all your body muscles peaceful, relaxed, and as soft as silk... Your legs become relaxed... Your arms and body trunk becomes peaceful and relaxed... The upper body muscles, especially around the chest, shoulders and neck, become quiet and relaxed... You make small abdominal inhalations... After inhalations, you just relax all body muscles completely to exhale air without efforts.

(***) This part between tree stars (located below) can be repeated several times.

... You can hear the waves... You can smell the ocean... The air is moist and warm... You feel a pleasant, cool breeze blowing from the ocean... You feel how the sun warms up your body... All muscles are quiet and relaxed... Your breathing is light... It almost disappears.

... You hear the rhythm of waves crashing to the shore... You smell the clean salt water and beach... You feel a comfortable light breeze and warm rays of the sun... Muscles are soft and quiet... All body is

Advanced Buteyko Breathing Exercises

relaxed... Inhalations are small... Exhalations are relaxed... You apply no efforts to exhale.

... You are enjoying peace and the warmness of the sun... You are enjoying the breeze... You are enjoying the waves... You feel calm, peaceful and relaxed... All your stresses melt away... Muscles are calmed and relaxed... Small abdominal inhalations and then total relaxation in order to exhale air passively.

(***) The part between tree stars (located above) can be repeated several times.

... Now you are ready to return back from your vacation... You do it slowly... In seconds, you will open your eyes and you will bring yourself back to your usual level of alertness and awareness, but you will keep the feeling of peace and relaxation and become energized.

... Open your eyes, stretch your arms and legs... You become fully alert... Muscles are refreshed... And your whole body is filled with energy.

You can use this script for breathing sessions of any intensity and as often as you wish. Visualization relaxation is a skill to be learned. If you practice the imagery of scenes more often, your skill will become stronger. Your muscles will be more relaxed, and breathing becomes even easier than after ordinary Buteyko breathing sessions.

Chapter 5. Breath holds and maximum pauses: health effects and uses

If you read his original writings, Dr. K.P. Buteyko often used the term "maximum pause" for the CP (Control Pause) or stress free breath holding time test done only until initial stress or discomfort. This fact may cause serious misunderstanding when Buteyko's words in Russian ("the maximum pause") are directly translated in English. The traditional Western and Russian meaning and definition of the "maximum pause" is breath holding for as long as possible and, if we are talking about the Buteyko method, all these breath holds are done after one's usual exhalation. For most people, including Buteyko students during their initial stages of learning, the maximum pause is about 2 times longer than the control pause, as we saw it above in the Buteyko Table of Health Zones.

Warning. Strong air hunger and similar effects can be produced during very shallow breathing (sometimes called "VSB") without any breath holds at all. This effect takes place when a student starts to breathe about twice less.

5.1 Maximum pauses, long breath holds and modern Buteyko teachers

The use of breath holds and extended breath holds (more than the CP) considerably varies among modern Buteyko teachers. Some Russian doctors did not and do not use any breath holds at all, while for followers of Sasha Stalmatsky, long breath holds and maximum pauses are very important or crucial parts of teaching the method. Furthermore, they often use AMP (absolute maximum pauses) which are done using special techniques, like the Valsalva maneuver (attempts to forcibly exhale while keeping the mouth and nose closed), fist clenching, stomping, jumping, etc. to prolong breath holding.

Unfortunately, due to poor knowledge of the method and the physiological effects of breath holds, some Buteyko practitioners may do more harm than good to certain groups of their students, while applying breath holds (see examples below).

5.2 Effects of maximum pauses and long breath holds on arteries and arterioles

There are many situations, when MP (Maximum Pauses) and AMP (Absolute Maximum Pauses) must not be done. Let us look at the causes of possible problems with long breath holds. Breath holding causes a fast rate of accumulation of CO_2 and reduction in O_2 in the lungs. Hence, the arterial blood gets more CO_2 and less O_2. Breath holding produces two opposite effects on the smooth muscles of blood vessels: vasodilation due to local hypercapnia and hypoxia, and central vasoconstriction caused by the release of norepinephrine and epinephrine that bind to alpha-receptors in most arterioles (in heart and skeletal muscles, epinephrine binding to beta-2 receptors causes vasodilation). Since norepinephrine and epinephrine are stress hormones, this vasoconstrictive effect is also influenced by psychological stress (in opposition to relaxation).

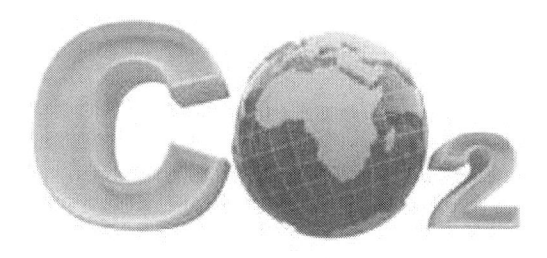

In the 1960's, when Dr. Buteyko was working in the respiratory laboratory, he and his colleagues conducted numerous studies about the effects of inhaled gases with various compositions on the tone of blood vessels. These results were published in several Soviet medical journals. He found that the body could maintain its physiological processes normally when changes in the composition of the inspired gas were gradual. Sudden changes in blood gases, as during breath holding, could lead to vasoconstriction and a significantly increased heart rate and blood pressure. In normal conditions, breath holding also causes the "diving reflex" when blood is diverted mainly to the brain and heart, and one's heart rate drops. In the case of vasoconstriction, it can last for many hours causing a maladaptive response to breath holding due to sudden changes in gas composition. As a result, the blood vessels can lose their sensitivity to CO2 and this can be a serious concern for some breathing students.

In order to achieve positive cardiovascular or circulatory effects, Dr. Buteyko taught his susceptible students how to gradually change their breathing without disruptive or sudden variations in blood gases. The reduced breathing exercise, without breath holds, was the main tool for ventilation reduction. These students practiced their breathing exercises with a light level of air hunger.

Now we can consider those situations when certain groups of people can experience various problems due to long pauses and sudden changes in the gas composition of the blood while practicing breathing exercises.

5.3 When and for whom long breath holds can cause problems

- In a person with hypertension, even the CP test results in increased blood pressure often, depending on the severity of the condition, and causes unpleasant symptoms. Such a practical result was received in many people with hypertension (i.e., Kohn & Cutcher, 1971). Moreover, some of them had a systolic blood pressure increase from about 200 to 260 mm Hg during maximum pauses, making the whole procedure of doing the maximum pause dangerous (Ayman & Goldshine, 1939). Indeed, in rare, but possible cases of an undetected serious organic defect in the heart muscle, the maximum pauses may cause severe complications, including physical damage to the heart muscle.

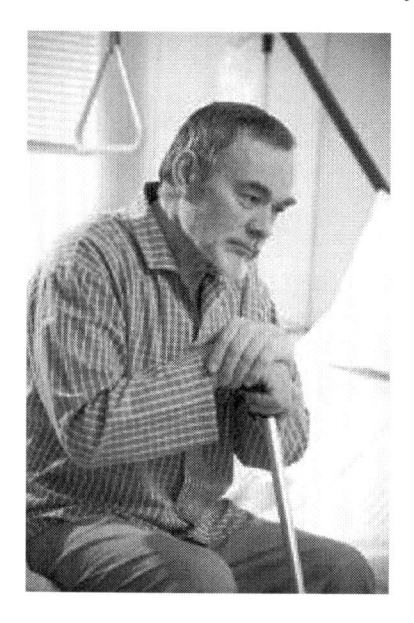

Warning. There are poorly educated Buteyko practitioners, who teach to their students with heart disease (e.g., hypertension) to practice maximum pauses and long breath holds, while producing these negative cardiovascular GI effects. Later, such students may have weeks or months of headaches, nausea, poor sleep, feeling weak, etc., while these practitioners sometimes mistakenly present these symptoms as a "cleansing reaction".

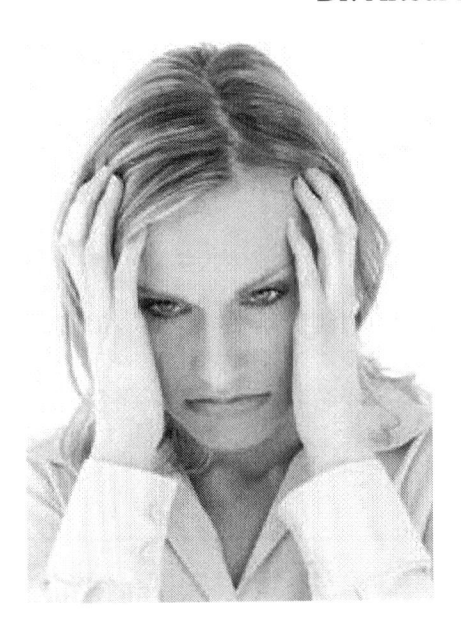

• Similar negative cardiovascular effects can lead to the appearance of migraine headaches in those people who are predisposed to this symptom.

• People with frequent panic attacks can experience their negative symptoms because of the CPs or longer pauses and mild or strong air hunger.

As another possible negative effect, long pauses and strong air hunger could cause a greatly increased blood flow due to hypercapnic vasodilation. As a result, people with some serious pathologies can experience negative symptoms. Here are several examples with this challenge:

• Many acute gastro-intestinal problems (gastritis, gastric ulcers, Crohn's disease and colitis (inflammatory bowel disease), intestinal ulcers, etc.) can dramatically worsen due to the suddenly incoming blood intensifying peristalsis. Flare-ups, opening of healed lesions, intensive wear of mucosal surfaces, causing such symptoms as gases, cramps, thirst, and diarrhea, all are possible complications.

Advanced Buteyko Breathing Exercises

• Patients with extensive damage to the kidneys' nephrons can experience so sudden an increase in blood flow to the kidneys, that the remaining working nephrons may be overburdened with the extra work to clean large amounts of the blood. Their possible congestion could result in the kidneys' failure with a sharp decrease in daily urinary output (i.e., less than 500 ml per day).

• Long breath holds can cause metastasis in people with malignant tumors (or cancer). Indeed, long pauses can be considered as light internal massage, due to their strong impact on microcirculation. Malignant cells can travel to neighboring lymph nodes, leading to the development of cancer in those people who do not increase their usual CPs. (Increase in the CP up to 35-40 s would indicate more normal work of the immune system and its ability to destroy malignant cells.)

• Patients with acute brain trauma will experience an increase in intracranial pressure (the pressure inside the skull). Moreover, should their blood have recently coagulated and therefore not yet formed a firm protective layer, this layer can be broken (due to larger pressure from underlying fluids) causing more bleeding and severe complications.

• Patients with recent bleeding cuts and other acute skin injuries will have dilation of small blood vessels and an increased blood flow. That will cause additional bleeding. If the cut or injury has just started to heal, opening of healed areas due to increased pressure from underlying blood layers is possible.

• A blood clot, due to thrombosis in the veins, can get loose and block a blood vessel leading to some organ causing severe problems or death.

• Maximum pauses, strong air hunger and high CPs (e.g., 30-35 s) can cause problems for people with transplanted organs due to an increased sensitivity of the immune system in relation to foreign cells leading to the rejection of donated organs.

- Spontaneous abortion of the fetus is possible, if the pregnant mother practices strong air hunger or long breath holds causing a large CP increase. The immune system, in case of serious initial toxicity of the fetus, may decide that it is easier to abort the fetus than to rebuild, repair and readjust the polluted tissues of the fetus.

References

Kohn RM & Cutcher B, *Breath-holding time in the screening for rehabilitation potential of cardiac patients*, Scandinavian Journal of Rehabilitative Medicine 1970; 2(2): p. 105-107.

Ayman D & Goldshine AD, *The breath holding test, a simple standard stimulus of blood pressure*, Archives of Internal Medicine 1939, 63: 899-906.

5.4 Cases with severe bleeding

In very rare situations (e.g., immediately after a dental or other surgery, or after a brain trauma, or after getting a bleeding cut) any breath holding, any sudden increase in carbon dioxide levels, or strong air hunger during RB could cause dilation of small blood vessels and increased bleeding.

Hyperventilation has another useful value in terms of survival of different animals. As it is known, arteries are hidden deeply under the skin in order to prevent bleeding, should a cut or severe open injury occur. Nature anticipated such an unlucky turn of events. Moreover, Nature also provided animals with hyperventilation in order to prevent excessive blood losses and possible death. There are medical studies that discovered that medical doctors could not draw a blood sample from the fingers of their patients who voluntarily hyperventilated. That was a normal result since low carbon dioxide values constrict the small blood vessels, hence, greatly reducing their blood flow.

One may notice that in natural conditions wild and domesticated animals and humans over-breathe when they have, for example, bleeding cuts. Such over-breathing is done unconsciously due to the pain and vision of their own blood. Later, after coagulation, the breathing is gradually reduced and the pain is also less. In addition, should any further bleeding occur, the emotional shock and vision of their own blood can again generate heavy over-breathing. This mechanism again helps to start the initial stages of wound healing.

However, any excessive carbon dioxide increase can immediately cause an opening of coagulated and hardened layers due to the higher pressure of the blood in the adjacent small vessels. That would result in additional blood losses.

The same ideas can be equally applied to the acute brain traumas. These considerations caused the wide-spread appearance of prophylactic hyperventilation in the medical practice of neurologists to prevent acute bleeding.

Therefore, should you get any bleeding wound or cut (after a surgery or injury, follow your natural impulses and breathe hard! That relates to the following situations with bleeding or severe hemorrhage:
- dental surgeries
- tonsillectomy
- operations on the brain, internal organs, and skin
- industrial and domestic accidents.

5.5 Loss of CO2 sensitivity

A loss of CO2 sensitivity due to a single breath hold (or a series of consecutive breath holds) depends on numerous factors, including the duration of breath holding, and hereditary (cardiovascular or hypertensive predisposition), life-style and environmental causes. Some of these predisposing factors are:
- being deprived of deep stages of sleep
- Ca deficiency
- insufficient protein and/or arginine in the diet
- overheating
- any inflammatory condition, including malignant and benign tumors.

There are also very rare situations (such as near death experiences, when carotid bodies removed, and when there is a denervation of respiratory muscles) leading to an abnormally long breath holding time.

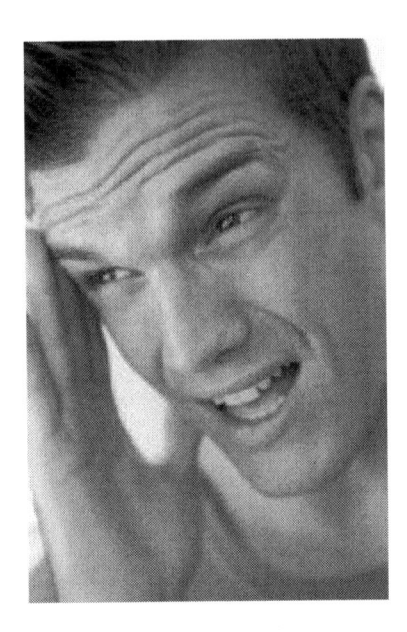

Generally, students with lower CPs and weak heredity in relation to the cardiovascular system have higher chances of developing this abnormal circulatory response (vasoconstriction) to breath holding. It is usually manifested in headaches or migraine-type sensations, feeling weaker, possible nausea, thirst on lips, etc. A short nap (even 3-5 minutes) can often eliminate the maladaptive response, but mild after-effects are going to last until the next night sleep. All other factors also play a role in this abnormal physiological reaction.

5.6 Other possible negative effects of maximum pauses or long breath holds

While one may not necessarily experience a loss of CO_2 sensitivity due to breath holding, many students, especially with low current CPs, can simply experience stress and an inability to control breathing after long breath holds even when they do not have any of the predisposing factors (panic attacks, hypertension, pregnancy, etc.) described above. But most of them would not experience any negative effects due to, for example, the Control Pause test.

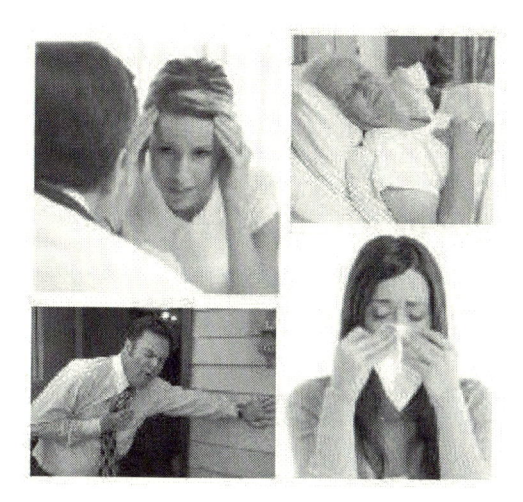

When the CP gets higher, the body's ability to tolerate maximum pauses and long breath holds gradually improves. Hence, longer breath holds can be practiced during later stages of learning (after some weeks or months of breathing training).

5.7 Common positive effects of maximum pauses or long breath holds

When the above cases are excluded, students can experience positive effects due to long breath holds. As it is also known among free divers, who are generally a healthy group of people, maximum breath holding has 4 stages: period of no respiratory sensations (the CP), period of struggle (from the CP to MP), period of bliss or euphoria due to the positive effects caused by the diving reflex (after the MP) and the last short period of new stress or more struggle. Such maximum breath holds, in experienced people, do not lead to severe overbreathing and stress later. They do not cause loss of CO_2 sensitivity. Furthermore, with some practice, students are able to practice reduced breathing or "switch" to reduced breathing after this one breath hold especially in cases, when they had hundreds or thousands shorter breath holds accompanied by reduced breathing later (the conditioned response due to past training).

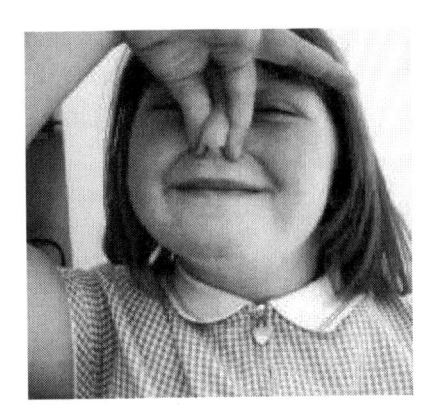

Hence, a certain training is required in order to consistently achieve these positive effects. While breathing sessions with strong air hunger and/or very long breath holds are most efficient for experienced breathing students, these sessions require an adaptation time and experience in order to achieve these positive effects.

5.8 How to check your reactions to maximum pauses and long breath holds

In most cases, student's personal sensations (or feelings) are correct indicators of bodily reactions and processes. Therefore, you can simply check how you feel after long breath holds and what the effects on your breathing patterns are.

In addition, in order to objectively check your cardiovascular responses, measure your heart rate (or pulse) some 2-3 minutes after the maximum pause or breath hold. If it is the same or even lower than prior to the breath hold, as it should be after Buteyko reduced breathing exercise (including very intensive reduced breathing sessions), your body accepts breath holding positively.

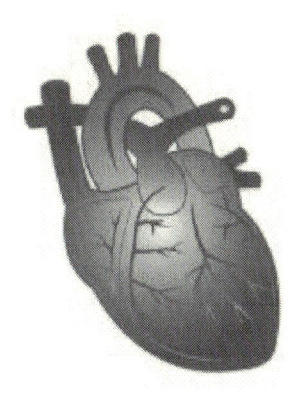

If your heart rate increases and remains high for many minutes (or hours) after the maximum pause or any other breath hold, you should not practice this breath hold. Instead, use more gentle versions of breathing exercises to improve your body-oxygen content and normalize your breathing.

Note that many groups of students (e.g., people with hypertension) may have adverse reactions even to a CP test. Such students should temporary avoid the CP test and there is a special daily log for them in the "Downloads" Section of NormalBreathing.com.

5.9 Summary of effects of breath holds

Depending on a variety of factors (health state, genetic factors, quality of sleep, morning CP, current health problems, ability to use the diaphragm at rest and during breath work, and many others), maximum pauses and other breath holds, even as short as one half of the CP, can cause various physiological reactions. In many cases, long pauses should not be used at all during initial stages of learning. As about the effects of long pauses and strong air hunger, cardiovascular responses play the main role in bodily circulatory adaptation to changes in blood gases. Measuring your own pulse and analyzing your body sensations help to prevent useless suffering, and damage to your own health.

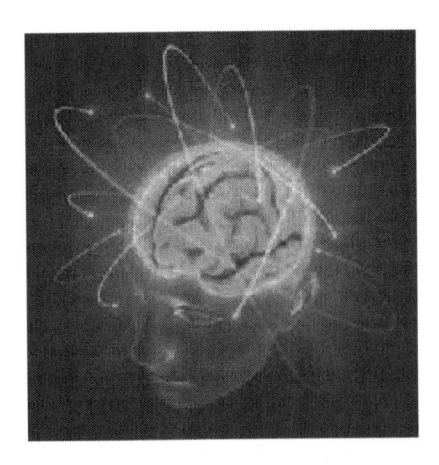

In nearly all cases, breathing students with over 30 s for their current CP can safely practice maximum pauses without any negative effects. However, most people with sufficient experience in reduced breathing (2-3 weeks) are also able to get benefits from extended and maximum pauses, even though they may only have about 15-20 s for their current CPs.

Chapter 6. Intensive Buteyko breathing exercises

It takes many hours of practice before the students can start using a moderate level of air hunger. Usually one can make this transition in about one-two weeks. Then some students can try more intensive sessions, for example, sessions with moderate air hunger.

During the RB (reduced breathing), it will be more difficult to relax since the higher CO2 increase will create conditions when the breathing center tries to make muscles tenser, while the goal of the student is to relax all muscles, especially the diaphragm.

6.1 How to create moderate or strong levels of air hunger

Breath holds create a desire to breathe more, and practice shows that students, if they start the RB after the CP, usually try to maintain the same level of air hunger during the RB (or a light level of air hunger) as they have at the end of the CP (i.e., first light comfortable air hunger).

The same effect is present after doing the EPs (extended pauses): the breathing students naturally generate moderate levels of air hunger during the RB after the EP. The EP can be, for example, 3, 5 or 10 s longer than the CP. While doing the initial EP, the student should also record and write down the CP. This means that you need to write in your daily log both facts: first, your CP and then the additional duration of breath holding.

For example, if you hold your breath for 20 seconds, but your CP (when the first desire to breathe took place) is 15 seconds, then you should write in your daily log: 15+5 s. This means that your CP was 15 s, but you held your breath for additional 5 seconds.

The same is true for breathing sessions with strong air hunger. If you hold your breath about twice as long as your current CP, then you will likely get strong air hunger (free divers may hold their breath for up to 3-4 times longer than their CPs when they try maximum breath holding). Then you can maintain the same strong air hunger during reduced breathing.

Of course, it is also possible just to do the CP test at the beginning of the session, but create moderate, strong or even very strong air hunger later, while doing the reduced breathing.

We are going to consider all these types of breathing exercises in this Chapter. In all these cases, you need to make sure that:
- these activities are safe for you
- you get benefits from these breathing exercises manifested in your improved wellbeing, lower pulse and increased final CPs.

Let us consider how we can apply these ideas for breathing exercises.

6.2 A breathing session with moderate intensity

After the RB and final pulse measurements, the student measures the CP, but continues to hold breath for an additional time, as long as 1/4 or 1/2 of the CP. For example, a student with 10 s CP can add 3, 4 or 5 seconds in order to have an EP (extended pause). If your CP is about 15 seconds, you can add 5-8 seconds to create a moderate air hunger. This is not your MP (maximum pause) yet, because nearly all people can hold their breath for as long as double the CP.

During the reduced breathing, in order to maintain moderate air hunger, you need to breathe about 20-30% less than you had before the session. A typical chart for reduced breathing with moderate air hunger is shown below.

Reduced breathing with medium air hunger

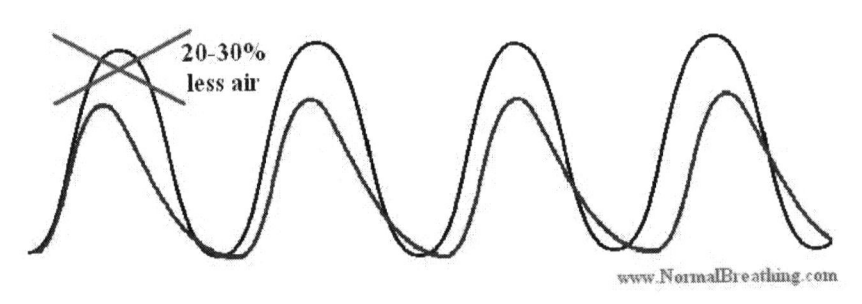

20-30% less air

www.NormalBreathing.com

Note that we do not count the breathing frequency during these exercises. It is more important to create a certain level of air hunger and good relaxation of body muscles.

The structure of such breathing sessions with moderate air hunger is the following:
Initial Pulse Test - Extended Pause (with CP recording) - RB (for 3-5 minutes)
- Intermediate Breath Hold (EP) - RB (for 3-5 minutes) -
....
- Intermediate Breath Hold (EP) - RB (for 3-5 minutes) -
- Intermediate Breath Hold (EP) - RB (for 3-5 minutes) - **Pulse Test - 2-3 Min Rest - Final CP Test**

Advanced Buteyko Breathing Exercises

The main goals for this type of session are the same as before: you need to be relaxed all the time and have small diaphragmatic (or abdominal) inhalations with relaxed exhalations. These sessions have the same criteria of success as for a single breathing session with light air hunger. You also need to apply the same criteria of success for the whole program related to your week-after-week overall progress.

When the breathing students, after 1-2 weeks of practicing light sessions, are provided with this choice (sessions with moderate air hunger), many of them prefer the sessions with moderate intensity since these students often find this new challenge (moderate air hunger with relaxation) interesting, challenging and more effective (in comparison with the sessions with light air hunger that were practiced during initial stages of learning).

A small number of students may still like sessions with light air hunger, when they have higher CPs and/or after weeks or even months of practice. These students may also get better results for light sessions.

If you record your sessions in your daily log, then you can analyze your sessions later and compare their effects so as to choose the more optimum sessions.

How to record moderate breathing sessions in the daily log

If you know how to record light sessions, recording breathing sessions with a moderate intensity is easy. There is only one small difference. Here is a daily log of a person who conducted several breathing sessions with a moderate degree of air hunger.

Date	Morn CP	Time (hour)	Initial pulse	Initial CP	Breath cycle or RB session time	Final pulse	Final CP	Physic. activity	Symptoms, medication and auxiliary activities
7.05	21	1 pm	70	22(+10)	24,30,32 - 16 m	66	28	55 min	fish oil - 1 tbs
		5 pm	68	20(+10)	23,28,34 - 16 m	66	29		
		11 pm	70	20(+10)	21,27,32 - 16 m	70	27		
8.05	20	9 am	70	22(+10)	24,28,29 - 16 m	68	28	60 min	fish oil - 1 tbs
		4 pm	74	24(+12)	22,23,30 - 16 m	70	29		
		10 pm	66	24(+12)	24,28,33 - 16 m	64	30		

For example, for the first breathing session from this daily log (at 1 pm on 7.05), the initial heart rate was 70. The initial CP was 22 seconds, but the student held his breath for additional 10 seconds ("+10" in the daily log). The durations of intermediate breath holds during reduced the breathing were 24, 30 and 32 seconds. The total duration of the breathing exercise was 16 minutes. (The session had 3 intermediate breath holds at 4, 8 and 12 minutes, or every 4 minutes.) The final pulse was 66 beats per minute, while the final CP was 28 seconds.

Using this simple idea (writing "+10" or some other number), it is easy to notice and evaluate (even weeks or months later) that this session had a moderate air hunger since the additional breath hold was about 50% (or half) of the CP.

The maximum duration of breathing sessions with a moderate air hunger is 25-30 minutes.

6.3 Intensive breathing sessions (with a strong air hunger)

Once you learned how to practice and progress with a moderate degree of air hunger (after about 1-2 weeks of practice), you can make the next step and start sessions with a strong air hunger. In order to naturally generate strong air hunger, we can apply the same approach as before. Do the MP (maximum pause), and then you can try to maintain the same level of shortage of air after this MP (i.e., strong air hunger). The main goals of such intensive breathing sessions are the same as before: you need to have good relaxation and breathe almost 2 times less (50%) than you breathed just before this breathing session.

It is possible to go further and do the MP and the RB with strong air hunger. The reader can apply the same ideas as in the previous section for sessions with moderate intensity.

The structure of the short session with strong intensity is:
Initial Pulse Test - Maximum Pause (with CP recording) - RB

(for 3-5 minutes)
- Maximum Breath Hold (MP) - RB (for 3-5 minutes) -
....
- Maximum Breath Hold (MP) - RB (for 3-5 minutes) -
- Maximum Breath Hold (MP) - RB (for 3-5 minutes) - End of the Reduced Breathing - Pulse Test - 2-3 Min Rest - Final CP Test

Here is an example of a breathing session that is 20 min long.

Breathing exercise with strong air hunger

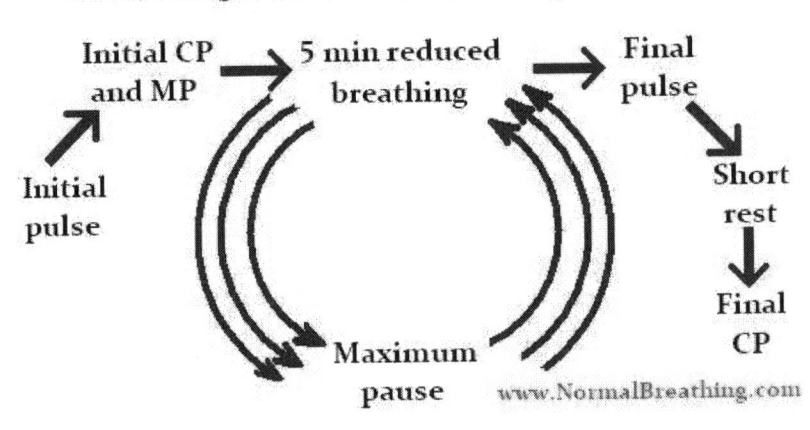

Initial CP and MP → 5 min reduced breathing → Final pulse

Initial pulse

Short rest

Maximum pause

Final CP

www.NormalBreathing.com

This session starts with the maximum pause but you need to measure and record your CP too. The session is based on cycles that include maximum pauses and reduced breathing with a strong degree of air hunger. Maximum pauses are done every 5 minutes. In total, the session involves 4 cycles and is 20 min long.

Note that 20 minutes is about the longest time for intensive sessions. Nearly all students will get negative effects of overtraining if they push themselves beyond 22-23 minutes. When the session goes beyond 20 minutes, their CPs sharply drop and heart rate increases. These effects are accompanied by feeling tired and even a possible headache. Breathing will become deregulated for some hours, and there are no positive effects of such sessions.

6.4 AMP and very intensive breathing sessions

Maximum Pauses are maximum breath holds that are done without any activities to prolong breath holding. We can hold breath longer if we start clinching out fists, or stomping the feet, or moving the shoulders, or nodding the head, or making swallowing movements that imitate inhalations. All these activities distract the breathing center and temporarily reduce air hunger. When we use these activities to hold our breath for as long as possible, we do AMPs (absolute maximum pauses).

AMPs cause even higher CO_2 levels in the lungs and the arterial blood (if the person does not suffer from COPD or ventilation-perfusion mismatch). Therefore, AMPs can be valuable to adapt and reset the breathing center to higher CO_2 values. The problem here is that positive effects of AMPs are likely to take place when the person is relaxed, and this is not easy for a novice. However, with experience in reduced breathing and doing pauses, relaxation is possible.

The structure of the short session with AMPs and very strong air hunger is:
Initial Pulse Test - Absolute Maximum Pause (with CP recording) - RB (for 3-5 minutes)
- Absolute Maximum Pause (AMP) - RB (for 3-5 minutes) -
- Absolute Maximum Pause (AMP) - RB (for 3-5 minutes) -
- Absolute Maximum Pause (AMP) - RB (for 3-5 minutes) - End of the Reduced Breathing - Pulse Test - 2-3 min rest - Final CP Test

Important warning. These very intensive sessions should be limited by 18 minutes and should not be practiced more than 1 time every 2 hours.

For advanced students and those who want to break through 40 s morning CP, sessions with a very strong air hunger are usually the most effective among all Buteyko exercises that are done at rest. Most students who have around 30-35 s for their initial CPs can get over 50 s CPs during or after these sessions. Some students get over 60 s for their final CPs. Obviously, this is an excellent result that demonstrates the high efficiency of intensive breathing sessions.

6.5 Sessions with variable breath holds and air hunger

Some breathing practitioners teach an additional type of intensive breathing exercises to their students. These breathing exercises involve a variable degree of air hunger. I rarely use these exercises for my students, but it is still good to know about this opportunity.

The most common type of these exercises involves a gradual increase in air hunger by doing breath holds of variable intensity. As a result of these breath holds, air hunger changes from light to very strong in the middle of the session. Then air hunger is reduced back to a light one.

The structure of such session is following:
Initial Pulse Test - CP Test - RB with light air hunger (for 3-5 minutes)
- Maximum Pause - RB with strong air hunger (for 3-5 minutes)
- Absolute Maximum Pause - RB with very strong air hunger (for 3-5 minutes) -
- Maximum Pause - RB with strong (or medium) air hunger (for 3-5 minutes) -
- Control Pause - RB with light air hunger (for 3-5 minutes) - End of the Reduced Breathing - Pulse Test - 2-3 min rest - Final CP Test

These sessions allow students to accumulate CO_2 more gradually in comparison with intensive and very intensive sessions. For these reasons, some students prefer and use these sessions in their practice.

Another option is to change the level of air hunger regardless of the duration of breath holds. For example, you can start with the CP only, but gradually reduce your air hunger from light to moderate levels, and then up to a strong or very strong air hunger. Then, in the middle of the session, you can have extended or maximum pauses with a strong or very strong air hunger. Then you can gradually reduce air hunger towards the end of the session.

6.6 The "click effect"

The "click effect" is a rare physiological phenomenon that takes place after very long breath holds in some students. This effect leads to an immediate transition to much easier breathing (almost without efforts) due to the adaptation of the breathing center to much higher CO_2 levels with a feeling or deep relaxation of body muscles accompanied by a sensation of very light comfortable breathing that does not cause air hunger. This effect allows a very fast nearly immediate CP improvement. The increase in one's CP can be up to 20-25 s. Here is an example.

Imagine a student with about 30-35 seconds for his current CP. If this student performs a very long breath hold, he is going to pass through the following stages:
- An easy part related to the CP (e.g., up to 30-35 seconds)
- A gradual increase in air hunger up to the maximum level at the end of the MP (from 30 to 60 seconds)
- Muscular movements in order to extent breath holding up to the AMP (absolute maximum pause) (from 60 to 90 seconds)
- Some super human will power that causes even longer breath holding (from 90 up to 110-120 seconds).

In this case, the total duration of this breath hold is about 2 minutes, and, at the end of this super long breath hold, this student experiences a light "click" that takes place in the head. After this click, the student releases the nose, but his first inhalation is naturally light, and he immediately notices that his breathing becomes very light, while his CP will often remain at over 50+ seconds even after night sleep (that will be about 4 hours long naturally).

Note that this situation is different from the situation during long breathing sessions, when a student gets 50+ or 60+ s for the final CP without the click effect. For some reasons, if the click effect does not take place, this student is likely to have a large CP drop at night, from 50+ seconds down to about 33-35 seconds (or smaller values) with more than 6 hours for his natural sleep.

The click effect has great benefits (nearly immediate transition through the most difficult threshold in breathing retraining - 40 s morning CP). However, less than half of all students (even with 30+ s CP) are able to experience the clock effect.

The effect was described in Russian Buteyko sources and there are some Western Buteyko students who experienced this effect too.

Too little information is known about this effect yet, and it seems that a variety of factors related to a good physiological state of the body can influence the appearance of this effect. Good sleep, good nutrition, a motivated state of mind, very relaxed muscles, grounding and some other factors favor, but do not guarantee the appearance of this effect.

6.7 Overtraining due to breathing exercises

The effect of overtraining due to breathing exercises is a rare phenomenon that occurs only in a small number of breathing students (probably less than 3-5%) due to too many long breath holds and too strong air hunger practiced for too long of a time.

As you may notice, the duration of breathing sessions has some limits. Even for light breathing sessions (with a light level of air hunger), there is a limit of about 35-40 minutes for a single session, while the next session can be done after 1.5-2 hours of rest. If these conditions are not fulfilled (for example, the breathing session is 50 min long or the next session is done after only 1 hour of rest), the breathing student can suffer the effect of overtraining.

How can one know that he or she gets overtrained? Let us consider an example. A person starts to practice a long session with a light air hunger. His initial CP and intermediate breath holds (during the

Advanced Buteyko Breathing Exercises

session) can have the following pattern:
- Initial CP: 20 s
- At 4 min: 15 s
- At 8 min: 17 s
- At 12 min: 20 s
- At 16 min: 22 s
- At 20 min: 23 s
- At 24 min: 22 s
- At 28 min: 24 s
- At 32 min: 25 s
- At 36 min: 24 s
- At 40 min: 25 s
- At 44 min: 11 s.

As you may notice, during the initial part of the session, the intermediate breath holds are shorter than the initial CP. Later, they become even larger than the initial CP. This pattern is very common when Buteyko exercises, with any degree of air hunger, are practiced correctly.

However, the main problem here is that the breath holds at 44 minutes is only 11 seconds. The drop from the previous number (25 seconds at 40 minutes) is more than 2 times.

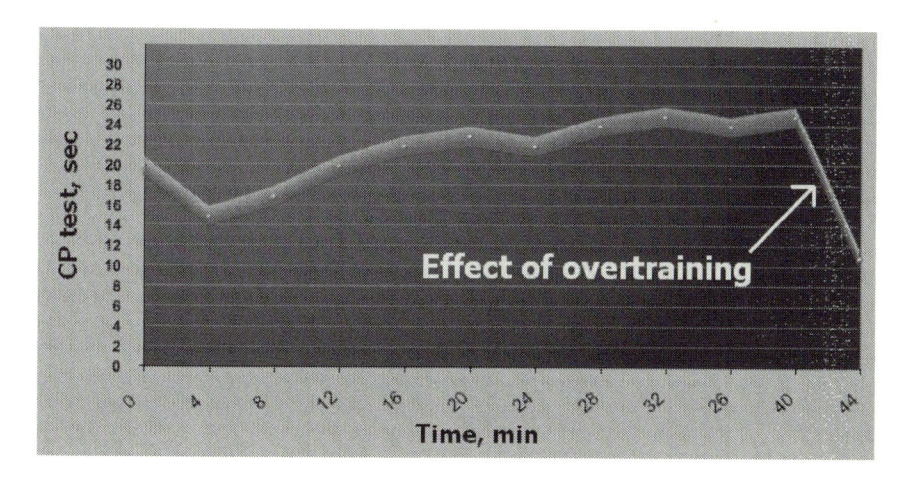

119

In such conditions with a sharp CP drop during the session, the student may get a slight air hunger and feel that there is something wrong with his breathing. Heart rate may increase or remain about the same.

Important. If you stop a breathing session at this exact moment (as soon as you see that your breath holds suddenly become too short in comparison with your previous numbers) and forget about breathing control, then you are likely to quickly recover and can have another session after 2 hours of rest. However, if you continue to have air hunger, you may suffer from more lasting symptoms that can easily lead to a loss of CO_2 sensitivity. Treatment of lost CO_2 sensitivity is considered in the last chapter of this book.

Ideally, you need to finish the breathing session slightly before this effect takes place. The guidelines provided in this book in relation to optimum duration of breathing sessions are created with some safety gap in order to prevent overtraining.

The effect of overtraining can take place during breathing sessions with a medium and strong air hunger as well. Therefore, durations of these breathing sessions are also restricted: for sessions with a moderate air hunger, by 25-30 minutes, and, for sessions with a strong air hunger, by 20 minutes. You also need a nearly 2 hours break between such sessions or practice them every 2 hours (e.g., you can start one breathing session at 6 pm and the next session at 8 pm).

If you practice beyond these limits or too often, you can become overtrained. For example, if your breathing session with a strong air hunger is 25 minutes long, you can experience the effect of overtraining. If you have only 1 hour break between two successive breathing sessions with maximum duration (e.g., you have two sessions with medium intensity 30 min each), then you can also suffer from temporary overtraining.

These are general guidelines since many other factors, such as a lack of sleep or deep stages of sleep, stress, nutritional deficiencies (especially calcium, EFAs, and arginine), and many other factors influence the onset and your ability to recover fast after you are overtrained. You can study these factors in more detail in the next Chapter (Chapter 7) since these factors are the same as for a loss of CO2 sensitivity.

6.8 Summary of intensive breathing exercises

For advanced students with 30+ s for their current CPs and for those people who have been practicing Buteyko breathing exercises for some weeks or even months, the sessions with strong and very strong air hunger are very effective. They allow them the achievement of higher CPs within a shorter period of time.

For those students who practiced breathing sessions for many months or even years, there is an additional effect that relates to the conditioning reflex. Each long breath hold leads to natural relaxation and easy breathing almost without effort. As we can see from these observations, diligent practice with hundreds, and sometimes thousands of sessions, pays back.

As a result of intensive sessions, the breathing student can spend less time on breathing exercises (while still pushing his or her CP up to 50+ s), and devote more time to, for example, physical exercise.

Physical exercise can also be combined with either basic breath control (such as paying attention that you have only nose breathing while working out), or with more sophisticated breathing exercises. We are going to consider them in the next Chapter.

Chapter 7. Treatment of blunted and lost CO2 sensitivity

This Chapter is devoted to treatment of a rare and difficult problem related to a loss of CO2 sensitivity. While less than 10% of breathing students suffer from this problem, it may not be easy to achieve success and easy breathing with low heart rate due to a variety of factors.

Most often, this problem appears in people with about 15-30 s CP. However, in very rare cases, a loss of CO2 sensitivity can be present in people with up to 50-60 s for the morning CP. In such extreme cases (at high CPs), a loss of CO2 sensitivity is manifested in abnormally high heart rate and appearance of headaches, while duration of sleep can be around 4 hours (or as expected).

7.1 Differences between blunted and lost CO2 sensitivity

Before finding the method to correct this problem and restore normal CO2 sensitivity of the respiratory center, let us consider differences between *blunted CO2 sensitivity* (also known as a condition with "blunted CO2 receptors") and *lost CO2 sensitivity*. These are different phenomena, and they require different solutions.

People with sleep apnea often suffer from a blunted CO2 sensitivity due to numerous apneic episodes (breath holds) that they experience during sleep. Since these people have heavy breathing before and after these breath holds, they do not get any positive effects or benefits from breath holds during sleep. As a result of this "training" during sleep, these people often have abnormally high CPs that do not corresponds with their breathing patterns.

For example, imagine two adults who have nearly the same breathing pattern at rest with the nearly same CO2 levels in the lungs. Assume that one of them has sleep apnea, while the second person does not have it. The person with sleep apnea may have up to 20-25 s for the CP test, while the second one has only about 15 s.

Now we can compare some parameters related to a blunted CO2 sensitivity with parameters that relate to a loss of CO2 sensitivity.

Parameters	Blunted CO2 sensitivity	Lost CO2 sensitivity
Expression of the effect	In a degree	"On" or "off" effect
Benefits from breath holds	Yes	No
Current goal	To increase the CP	To restore CO2 sensitivity
Can benefit from reduced breathing?	Yes	No
Final pulse (after breathing sessions)	Gets lower	Gets higher
Heart rate at rest (sitting)	70-90	Very high (90+)

Note that this Table provides only the general picture. For example, if one has over 90 beats per minute for pulse rate at rest, this does not mean that this person has lost his or her CO2 sensitivity. Many people with a severe form of heart disease (and with less than 10 s CP) often have over 100 beats per minute for their resting pulse.

7.2 Treatment of blunted CO2 sensitivity

Since people with blunted CO2 sensitivity can get immediate and long-term benefits from Buteyko breathing exercises, they can have breathing sessions as described in this book while following usual restrictions and contraindications. Therefore, they can gradually increase their air hunger levels.

With easier breathing during sleep and higher morning CPs, people with sleep apnea gradually have fewer apneic episodes during sleep and with more than 25-30 s for their morning CPs, their breathing pattern during sleep becomes normal with presence of deep stages of sleep and disappearance of symptoms of sleep apnea during the day.

The situation with those who use CPAP machines can be different depending on one's ability to change machine ventilation parameters and other factors.

Treatment of lost CO2 sensitivity can be divided into 2 stages:
Stage 1. Restoration of CO2 sensitivity.
Stage 2. Restoration of normal body response to breath holds and air hunger.

7.3 Restoration of normal heart rate

During Stage 1, the key factor that a person needs to target is his or her heart rate with the goal being to get it below 80 beats per minute. The person should not be involved in any breath holds or practice reduced breathing. They will worsen the problem by getting increased headache and higher pulse rate. It is also necessary to pay attention to any other factors that causes worsened symptoms and increased heart rate.

Once CO2 sensitivity is lost, these parameters need to be addressed:

- **Sleep and deep stages of sleep** are among the most effective factors to restore lost CO2 sensitivity. In most cases, even a five minute nap during the day is able to immediately reduce heart rate below 80 beats per minute and normalize breathing control by the breathing center. Similarly, night sleep usually leads to recovery of

Advanced Buteyko Breathing Exercises

CO2 sensitivity. However, if deep stages of sleep are absent, it is very easy to lose CO2 sensitivity again due to a very short breath hold, mild overheating, stress, and many other factors. Note that overheating during sleep (for example, due to too warm blankets) can prevent restoration of CO2 sensitivity even during sleep.

- **Physical exercise** with nose breathing only, but without breath holds and without breathing control, assists your progress. Some people can restore CO2 sensitivity after one session of physical activity with the factor that is described next.

- **Relaxation of body muscles** with no breath holds and no air hunger is an excellent exercise. In rare cases, good relaxation with slow deep breathing and/or humming or with no breathing control, in a cool environment, can restore CO2 sensitivity within 5-10 minutes.

- Avoid **allergy triggers** since they dramatically increase chances of lost CO2 sensitivity.

- **Humming** (after meals or nearly all the time) helps to increase production and utilization of nasal nitric oxide and sometimes can restore CO2 sensitivity in 5-20 minutes.

- Make sure that you have **no air hunger and no breath holds**.

- **Surrounding temperature** (no overheating or overcooling) is very important. In some people, overheating can be the major trigger of lost CO2 sensitivity.

- Prolonged and/or very **cold shower and cold air baths** are often able to restore lost CO2 sensitivity in a matter of minutes. This makes sense since colder conditions naturally push the blood from veins, which are located on the surface of the human body, into arteries that are deeply hidden. This is exactly what the body needs: expansion of arteries and lower heart rate.

- **Earthing** prevents and reduces inflammation. This is another essential factor that can play a crucial role in some people. It is particularly important for people with sleeping problems or poor sleep, inflammation and problems that relate to muscle and nerve cells. For more information about Earthing, search online or visit the relevant Module on the website NormalBreathing.com with grounding techniques provided.

- **Essential fatty acids** are effective to reduce inflammation, especially for people with less than 20 s CP.

- **Arginine in diet** (to increase nitric oxide production) helps to dilate arteries and arterioles. This effect directly counteracts the main symptom of lost CO_2 sensitivity: constricted arteries and arterioles.

- Additional **calcium supplementation**, even above the recommended amounts, will help to keep the nerve and muscle cells, including the smooth muscles around arteries and arterioles in a health relaxed state.

- **Correct posture** provides more oxygen for the blood and increases one's CP.

- Avoid **too low and too high blood glucose levels** since both these factors can become triggers of lost CO_2 sensitivity.

Any additional lifestyle risk factor will make your symptoms worse. For example, **mouth breathing** will increase your heart rate. **Supine sleep** may be beneficial if it is very short (i.e., you take a 5-min nap on your back). However, sleeping on your back at night will restore lost CO_2 sensitivity, but will also cause your low morning CP. Therefore, it is better to follow standard guidelines related to best sleeping positions for sleeping at night.

Addressing all these factors should lead to a quick restoration of lost CO_2 sensitivity. This is manifested in lower heart rate at rest (less than 80 beats per minute while sitting) and disappearance of the chronic headache.

7.4 Restoration of normal CO_2 sensitivity

Advanced Buteyko Breathing Exercises

The second stage of treatment of lost CO_2 sensitivity is to adjust the body so that it has normal (or positive) responses to breath holds and air hunger. In other words, the body should be repaired to the state when it can have a positive reaction to breathing exercises.

If a person has good sleep and addresses all the factors described above, then he or she can try to practice reduced breathing in 2-3 days after restoration of CO_2 sensitivity.

People with severe sleeping problems may need more time before they can safely practice reduced breathing and, later, other breathing exercises. In such cases, they need to focus on crucial sleep factors, such as grounding during sleep, sleeping on a hard bed or floor, good air quality, going for a walk in fresh air (before sleep), and many other practices of the Buteyko breathing method. Such people may require some weeks before they can get benefits from and resume breathing exercises. When this process of recovery is slow, they can try to have one session of reduced breathing (for about 10-12 minutes) and measure its effects on their pulse. Once their final pulse (after the session) gets lower than the initial pulse, they can increase the number and duration of sessions, but still without breath holds.

The next step is to resume those breathing exercises that include the CP test, while monitoring one's symptoms, heart rate, and the CP changes after breathing exercises.

More intensive breathing exercises should also be started gradually following the same rules outlined above. First, monitor your body's reaction to sessions with a moderate degree of air hunger. In 3-4 days, you can try breathing exercises with a moderately strong degree of air hunger. Some days later, if you achieve success during your past breathing sessions, you can proceed to the most demanding or most intensive breathing exercises.

Chapter 8. Breathing exercises during physical activity

Breathing exercises during physical activity need to be carefully tailored to the current health state, fitness, recent training, and the CP of the breathing student. For most people and in most situations, the CP is the main parameter that defines their optimum program of breathing exercises during working-out. In other words, your CP tells you which breathing exercises you can safely and effectively use in order to move forward. This is also true when you combine physical exercise with breathing sessions.

However, it is very important to increase duration and intensity of exercise gradually since too many breathing students get higher CPs (e.g., over 30 seconds) feeling very powerful and energetic (sometimes as never before in their lives) and they do too intensive sessions for too long time causing injuries to muscles, tendons and ligaments.

Apart from the gradualness idea, there are several groups of people who cannot exercise to the normal extent due to their health problems. Let us start with these people who have restrictions and limitations to their ability to exercise.

8.1 Restrictions and limitations

These groups of people require adjustments to their physical activity.

People with COPD

This idea (that your CP is the key factor) is not applicable for people with COPD (chronic obstructive pulmonary disease), severe bronchitis and emphysema included. They need to restore their lungs, often up to 90% or higher functional lung capacity, before they can follow the program outlined below. Even with about 90% of lung capacity, these people still need to take exercise much easier than ordinary people.

As a result, the main type of physical exercise for most people with COPD is walking, while the main breathing exercise during walking is breathing only through the nose (in and out). This is true even when they get up to 35 s CP. At this stage, when they keep their CPs above 30 s and do not cause additional damage to their lungs, there is a gradual and steady improvement in their lungs and lung function tests (due to restoration of alveoli) leading to improved tolerance to exercise (with nose breathing).

People with musculoskeletal and neurological problems

People with some serious degenerative health problems, such as severe arthritis, multiple sclerosis, Parkinson's disease and others, are often limited in their ability to exercise. Even though improved CPs of many of such breathing students greatly boost their energy levels and desire to exercise, they need to pay close attention to their symptoms and body signs while doing any physical exercise. Pain in muscles, bones, tendons, and ligaments is nearly always a sign to stop exercise or reduce its intensity.

People with ulcers and IBD (inflammatory bowel disease)

People with serious digestive problems, which also include ulcerative colitis and Crohn's disease, can worsen their GI health and even produce exacerbations or digestive flare-ups due to wrong types of physical exercise. For example, bending forward and squatting increase pressure on digestive organs and can trigger intensive peristaltic waves, in such people, leading to GI flare-up.

As a result, this group of people need to find those types of exercise that are suitable for their current health state and do not trigger typical symptoms of GI exacerbations, such as ear buzzing, unquenchable thirst on lips, frequent urination, increased soiling (with the need to use more toilet paper), cold feet, and others. You can find more detail about special adjustments required for some people with digestive problems in the PDF book "How to Improve Digestion with Lifestyle and Higher Body O2" or in the Kindle book "Crohn's Disease and Colitis: Hidden Triggers and Symptoms".

8.2 Breathing techniques during exercise for people with various CP ranges

People with very low current CPs (less than 10 s)

Restoration of normal breathing (that corresponds to about 40 s CP) is often a difficult, or sometimes impossible, without physical exercise. When the CP is very low (less than 10 s), many breathing students, especially with prolonged chronic diseases, can practice only breathing exercises since nearly any physical activity is usually too difficult. During exercise, such people often start mouth breathing even while walking slowly or with a normal speed. People with cardiovascular problems can experience acute exacerbations, and have heart attacks and strokes due to physical exercise leading to overexertion.

Instead of walking, they can use easy stretching exercises for the legs, arms, spine, and neck. All types of physical exercise should be done with only nasal breathing. These very easy forms of physical activity increase circulation and improve lymphatic drainage. Nose breathing (in and out) is the main breathing exercise or requirement for all people with very low CPs.

However, after practicing breathing exercises, these people are able to get more than 10 s CP. In fact, Dr. Buteyko invented reduced breathing, which is the main Buteyko breathing exercise, for these severely sick people with very low CPs. His intention was to increase their CPs to higher levels, so as to allow these patients to exercise physically and further move their CPs up.

If you are able to walk without creating more symptoms and health problems, while breathing only through the nose, then you can do walking and other types of exercise, but with nose breathing (in and out) only. This will be a great assisting factor in your CP growth.

People with low current CPs (between 10 and 20 s)

Advanced Buteyko Breathing Exercises

At this point of their health journey (when their CP is between 10 and 20 seconds), it is very useful, for further CP progress, to include easy or light types of physical exercise. For example, one can start walking on an even surface (without steep up-hills that can cause shortness of breath and mouth breathing).

When the current CP is around 10-14 seconds, the speed of walking generally should be slow. At these CP levels (10 to 14 s), tolerance to exercise is very poor. Once these people get up to 16-18 s CP, they can walk faster while breathing only through the nose.

At about 18-20 s CP, most people are able to exercise using power walking, and slow uphill walking (provided that incline is not too steep). The main requirement for breathing students with such CPs (18-20 s) is the same as before (nose breathing only). But at this stage, it is possible to practice reduced breathing or deliberately restrict ventilation during physical exercise. In addition, people with about 18-20 s for their current CPs are also able to combine physical activity with a very powerful breathing exercise that I call "**Steps for Adults**". This exercise is explained below.

As for the previous situation (less than 10 s), this zone (10-20 s for the current CP) also has some exceptions. Some people (probably fewer than 5%) are able to do jogging or running with nose breathing even when they have less than 20 s for their current CP. If this is the case for you, then you can do these and other types of more intensive exercise.

People with medium CPs (between 20 and 30 s)

Most people with over 20 s CP are able to start jogging. In fact, Soviet and Russian Buteyko doctors insisted that their patients started more active types of exercise with nose breathing only (in and out) as soon as their current CPs were above 20 s. In nearly all cases, this CP breakthrough (to 20+ seconds) occurs after breathing sessions. It is not necessary, but useful, for people with medium CPs, to practice two simple breathing exercises during physical activity. These respiratory exercises are provided below.

People with 30-40 s CP

Breathing students get most benefits from breathing exercises during physical exercise when they have 30-40 s for their current CP. At this stage, it is much easier to manipulate breathing during workouts. Such people can easily have short breath holds while exercising. In addition, most of them already have experience in practicing reduced breathing at rest. Therefore, they are able to practice reduced breathing during light or even moderate exercise.

People with over 40 s for the morning CP

Students who have more than 40 s for their morning CP can practice reduced breathing with longer breath holds (up to 10 s and more) even during very intensive exercise. In fact, it is relatively easy for them since breathing students with such high CPs enjoy and crave physical exercise naturally.

8.3 Exercise 1. Breath holds and reduced breathing during physical exercise

Practicing reduced breathing and doing breath holds during intensive types of exercise (such as jogging) greatly amplify the effects of physical exercise. However, your ability to practice these types of breathing exercises during physical activity depends on exercise intensity. There is no need to do exercise at maximum intensity. In fact, it is possible to get more benefits from exercise if you exercise at slightly lower intensity (than your maximum intensity with nose breathing). Easier exercise provides a person with more flexibility in breathing control: it is easier to practice short breath holds (e.g., about 5 seconds) and reduced breathing while exercising.

Why is it so? At highest intensity levels, you will be only focused on having nasal breathing. With slightly lower intensities, you will be able to do much more with your breathing than just nose breathing.

What exactly can be done? Every 2 minutes, while for example running, do short breath holds (about 5 s or longer if you have good

Advanced Buteyko Breathing Exercises

CPs), and practice reduced breathing after these breath holds. You can practice this simple breathing technique for as long as you exercise.

You may remember that when we do breathing exercises at rest, there is a certain time limit for such sessions. Intensive breathing sessions at rest are limited to about 18-20 minutes. If you practice breathing exercises longer than 20 minutes with a strong or very strong air hunger, you can overtrain. The duration of intermediate breath holds will sharply drop down to about 1/2 of previous numbers, and you will feel worse with a possible headache.

However, intensive physical exercise offers some additional positive factors in comparison with sitting at rest, such as high heart rates, perspiration and muscular work. All these factors favor easier adaptation of the human body to higher CO_2 levels. In other words, exercise with breath holds and reduced breathing is a more natural activity for humans than sitting and practicing intensive breathing exercises.

8.4 Exercise 2. "Steps for Adults"

This is one of the most effective breathing exercises to boost CO_2 to higher levels. It can be started when one's CP is about 18 s or higher. People with COPD and other problems that cause hypoxemia or low blood oxygenation require higher CP numbers in order to use and get benefits from this exercise.

This exercise is particularly effective for students with diabetes and reactive hyperglycemia. Applying this exercise helps to reduce too high blood sugar in minutes.

This breathing exercise is for advanced students. This means that, before doing this exercise, you need to accumulate some experience. Learn how to practice reduced breathing with a moderate or strong level of air hunger and good relaxation of muscles for some days, or better 2-3 weeks. Then you can transfer your experience from breathing sessions at rest to breathing sessions during light physical exercise, such as walking.

Instructions

You start "Steps for Adults" exercise with walking while pinching the nose and holding your breath. Do it until you get a moderate or strong air hunger. Then you release your nose and make sure that your first inhalation is only through the nose. This first inhalation is going to be big. However, immediately after this deep inhalation, you need to practice reduced breathing while walking for the next 1-3 minutes.

You are going to notice that, while you do reduced breathing, air hunger gradually disappears. It usually takes about 2 minutes. Then you do another breath hold and create another CO_2 boost. After you finish the second breath hold, you repeat the same actions: the first large inhalation through the nose, and then reduced breathing with air hunger and good muscular relaxation.

As a result of repetitive breath holds with reduced breathing, you keep your CO_2 levels very high all the time.

Remember about good relaxation of all body muscles. Keep chest muscles relaxed too. Make inhalations using the diaphragm (or abdominal muscles). It is common that you will find it difficult to keep the diaphragm relaxed, as it happens during reduced breathing at rest. Your goal will be the same: make small abdominal inhalations, relax to exhale and keep the diaphragm relaxed.

You can periodically shake your arms and shoulders for better relaxation of the upper body.

Therefore, this exercise has the following structure:
- **While Walking All the Time, You Do:**
- **Breath Holding (until a moderate or strong air hunger) - Reduced Breathing for 1-3 min**
- **Breath Holding (until a moderate or strong air hunger) -**

Advanced Buteyko Breathing Exercises

**Reduced Breathing for 1-3 min
- Breath Holding (until a moderate or strong air hunger) -
Reduced Breathing for 1-3 min**

....
....

**.- Breath Holding (until a moderate or strong air hunger) -
Reduced Breathing for 1-3 min**

For the first several days, do this exercise with a moderate degree of air hunger. Later, you can proceed to strong and very strong degrees of air hunger.

The maximum duration of the exercise with strong air hunger is 18 minutes and with moderate air hunger is about 20-22 minutes.

Record this exercise in your daily log

These sessions can be recorded in a daily log. This is especially important for progressing students or those learners who move their CPs up. In order to record the "Steps for Adults" session, after 5-7 min of rest, while sitting, measure your initial heart rate and the initial CP. Then do the exercise as it is described above.

The middle column of the daily log is used for the duration of intermediate breath holds (when you do reduced breathing at rest) and for the total duration of the session. When recording information about the "Steps for Adults" session, you can record the number of steps that you make during this exercise, and its total duration.

After you finish the exercise, you need to sit and rest for about the same duration of time as the duration of this exercise. Then you can measure your final CP and pulse. For example, if you do this exercise for 15 minutes, you need about 15-20 minutes of rest. Then you can measure your final parameters.

If you measure your final parameters immediately after the exercise, you will not get the numbers that reflect your new health state. The

CP is going to be shorter, and the heart rate remains high for many minutes after the session.

Here is an example of the daily log with two "Steps for Adults" sessions. These sessions are outlines on the following picture.

Advanced Buteyko Breathing Exercises

Date	Morn CP	Time (hour)	Initial pulse	Initial CP	Breath cycle or RB session time	Final pulse	Final CP	Physic. activity	Symptoms, medication and auxiliary activities
7.05	21	1 pm	70	22(+10)	24,30,32 - 16 m	66	28	55 min	fish oil - 1 tbs
		5 pm	68	20(+10)	23,28,34 - 16 m	66	29		
		11 pm	70	20(+10)	21,27,32 - 16 m	70	27		
8.05	20	9 am	70	22(+10)	24,28,29 - 16 m	68	28	60 min	fish oil - 1 tbs
		4 pm	74	24(+12)	22,23,30 - 16 m	70	29		
		10 pm	66	24(+12)	24,28,33 - 16 m	64	30		
9.05	23	8 am	72	22	S: 16,12,14,16-12	60	29	60 min	fish oil - 1 tbs
		5 pm	72	23(+12)	21,23,31 - 16 m	70	31		Steps
		9 pm	74	24	S: 14,13,15,20-12	62	32		
		11 pm	68	22(+12)	20,24,30 - 16 m	66	30		

We can see that the first Step session was done at 8 am on May 9th. The initial pulse was 72 beats per minute and the initial CP 22 seconds. The numbers of pairs of steps (for the daily log, we count the number of pairs of steps) were 16, 12, 14, and 16 pairs of steps. The session was 12 minutes long and the breath holds were done at 0, 3, 6, and 9 minutes or every 3 minutes.

After the session the student has a rest of 15 minutes that is not reflected in this log. Then the final parameters were measured: 60 beats per minute for the final pulse (but we measure the pulse during 30 seconds, and then multiply it by 2), and 29 seconds for the final CP.

Other effects related to this exercise

Many students get very low heart rates after "Steps for Adults". Many of my students achieved their record lowest numbers for their heart rates. This means that they never had such low heart rates before. If this is the case, these students require more physical exercise since this great result (ever lowest heart rates) indicates that their cardiovascular system responds very well to this combined exercise.

Are there any particular groups of people who can get the most benefits from this exercise? This exercise can become the most effective and most frequently used breathing exercise for people with sedentary lifestyle or with professional jobs that require computer work and/or sitting. In this case, during breaks, students need to make a decision. Should they do breathing exercises or physical exercise? The exercise "Steps for Adults" allows us to combine both exercises and get benefits from both activities.

8.5 Breathing devices for physical exercise

Breathing devices, strictly speaking, were never endorsed by Dr. Buteyko. However, had Dr. Buteyko measured physiological effects of Training Mask on breathing using his combine (a complex that

Advanced Buteyko Breathing Exercises

measured over 30 body parameters in real time), he surely would have approved and maybe even liked this device.

For students with higher current CPs (over 20 s at least, but better over 30 s), the most effective form of physical exercise involves the use of Training Mask. Training Mask doubles the dead volume (the amount of air that is inhaled but does not participate in gas exchange) in comparison with nose breathing. Here is a chart with numbers:

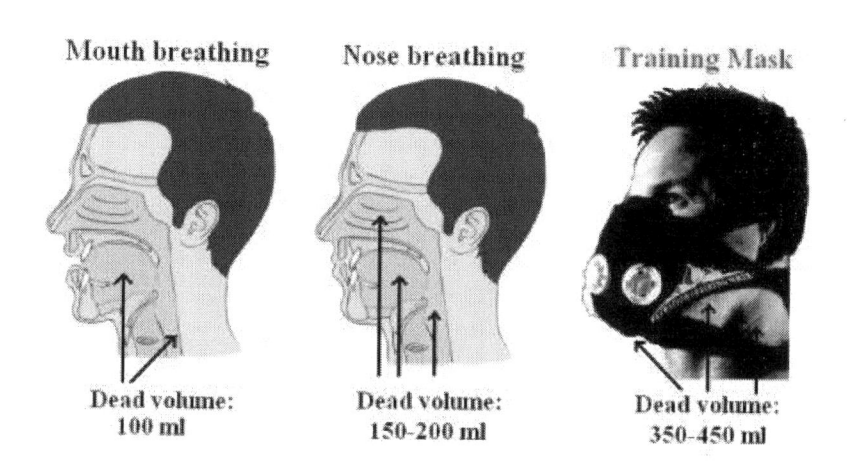

Mouth breathing	Nose breathing	Training Mask
Dead volume: 100 ml	Dead volume: 150-200 ml	Dead volume: 350-450 ml

In addition, Training Mask provides increased resistance to breathing, and this resistance can be suitably adjusted in a wide range of parameters. This is easy to achieve: just replace one or both valves with plastic holes. The number of holes in one plastic cap is 1, 2 or 4. As a result, Training Mask can mimic effects of high altitude from 3,000 feet up to 18,000 feet (or from about 1 to 6 km).

As a result of these two factors (increased dead volume and increased resistance), there are several positive effects of Training Mask during exercise:
- much easier adaptation to higher CO_2 and lower O_2 while exercising
- powerful stimulation of the diaphragm
- intensive drainage of the lymph nodes located under the diaphragm and stimulation of internal organs due to a large amplitude of

changes in internal pressure during inhalations/exhalations
- nearly natural nasal breathing during exercise
- very fast recovery after workouts.

In fact, the longer you exercise, the better the adaptation. This is not the case when you exercise with nose breathing. It is known that long session of physical exercise, even with breath control, require many hours for the CP to recover. For most breathing students, the positive effect of 2+ hours of good physical exercise is reflected only on the next morning CP. However, with Training Mask, the recovery is nearly immediate. Once you finish working out and remove the mask, there is no desire to overbreathe. Training Mask provides nearly instantaneous adaptation to higher CO2.

For the full review of the Training Mask, comments, and testimonials, visit http://www.normalbreathing.com/d/training-mask.php.

Conclusions

People use Buteyko breathing exercises for different purposes.

Many experienced students apply Buteyko exercises just to maintain their health and current CPs. This is a relatively simple and stress-free situation. Other breathing students try to get higher CP numbers. While they move forward, everything works OK since these students experience numerous positive changes due to slower and easier breathing with higher CPs. The problems and stress arise when these aspiring students get stuck.

This is the most frequent topic in emails and messages from other sources that I get from practicing breathing students, nearly always new people from whom I have never heard from before. Experience shows that, in most cases, these students should try a 2-3 day test. During this test, they need to increase the total amount of breathwork to about 2 hours per day and get more physical exercise as well. This will help the student to check the possible source of resistance of the body in relation to easier breathing and higher CPs. There are 2 general outcomes for this test:

1. If this student is able to get larger CPs, it is likely that this student can remain at this higher CP level even with slightly reduced parameters of his work. The source of resistance, whatever it was, has been eliminated using this test.

2. If this student remains at about the same CP, he or she needs to dig for other causes of resistance, such as focal infections (root canals included).

Using personally tailored Buteyko breathing exercises greatly facilitates smoother and easier progress. I hope that this book helps you to solve this challenge, and that you found this book useful for your practice.

Dr. Artour Rakhimov

If you have questions, suggestions and/or concerns related to this book, feel free to leave a comment on the main website.

All the best and easier breathing, Dr. Artour Rakhimov.

About the author: Dr. Artour Rakhimov

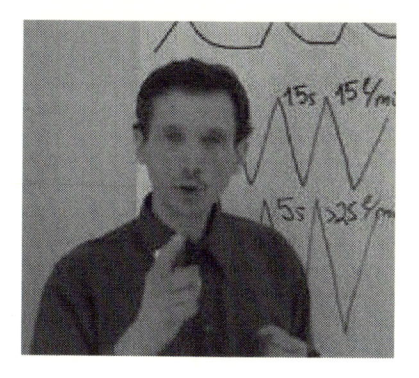

* High School Honor student (Grade "A" for all exams)
* Moscow University Honor student (Grade "A" for all exams)
* Moscow University PhD (Math/Physics), accepted in Canada and the UK
* Winner of many regional competitions in mathematics, chess and sport orienteering (during teenage and University years)
* Good classical piano-player: Chopin, Bach, Tchaikovsky, Beethoven, Strauss (up to now)
* Former captain of the ski-O varsity team and member of the cross-country skiing varsity team of the Moscow State University, best student teams of the USSR
* Former individual coach of world-elite athletes from Soviet (Russian) and Finnish national teams who took gold and silver medals during World Championships
* Total distance covered by running, cross country skiing, and swimming: over 100,000 km or over 2.5 loops around the Earth
* Joined Religious Society of Friends (Quakers) in 2001
* Author of the publication which won Russian National 1998 Contest of scientific and methodological sport papers
* Author of the books, as well as an author of the bestselling Amazon books:
 - *"Oxygenate Yourself: Breathe Less" (Buteyko Books; 94 pages; ISBN: 0954599683; 2008; Hardcover)*
 - *"Cystic Fibrosis Life Expectancy: 30, 50, 70, ..." 2012 - Amazon Kindle book*

Dr. Artour Rakhimov

- "Doctors Who Cure Cancer" 2012 - Amazon Kindle book
- "Yoga Benefits Are in Breathing Less" 2012 - Amazon Kindle book
- "Crohn's Disease and Colitis: Hidden Triggers and Symptoms" 2012 - Amazon Kindle book
- "How to Use Frolov Breathing Device (Instructions)" - 2012 - PDF and Amazon book (120 pages)
- "Amazing DIY Breathing Device" - 2010-2012 - PDF and Amazon book
- "What Science and Professor Buteyko Teach Us About Breathing" 2002
- "Breathing, Health and Quality of Life" 2004 (91 pages; Translated in Danish and Finnish)
- "Doctor Buteyko Lecture at the Moscow State University" 2009 (55 pages; Translation from Russian with Dr. A. Rakhimov's comments)
- "Normal Breathing: the Key to Vital Health" 2009 (The most comprehensive world's book on Buteyko breathing retraining method; over 190,000 words; 305 pages)

* Author of the world's largest website devoted to breathing, breathing techniques, and breathing retraining (www.NormalBreathing.com)
* Author of numerous YouTube videos (http://www.youtube.com/user/artour2006)
* Buteyko breathing teacher (since 2002 up to now) and trainer
* Inventor of the Amazing DIY breathing device and numerous contributions to breathing retraining
* Whistleblower and investigator of mysterious murder-suicides, massacres and other crimes organized worldwide by GULAG KGB agents using the fast total mind control method
* Practitioner of the New Decision Therapy and Kantillation
* Level 2 Trainer of the New Decision Therapy
* Health writer and health educator

Printed in Great Britain
by Amazon.co.uk, Ltd.,
Marston Gate.